The Xingyi Quan
of the Chinese Army

# The Xingyi Quan of the Chinese Army

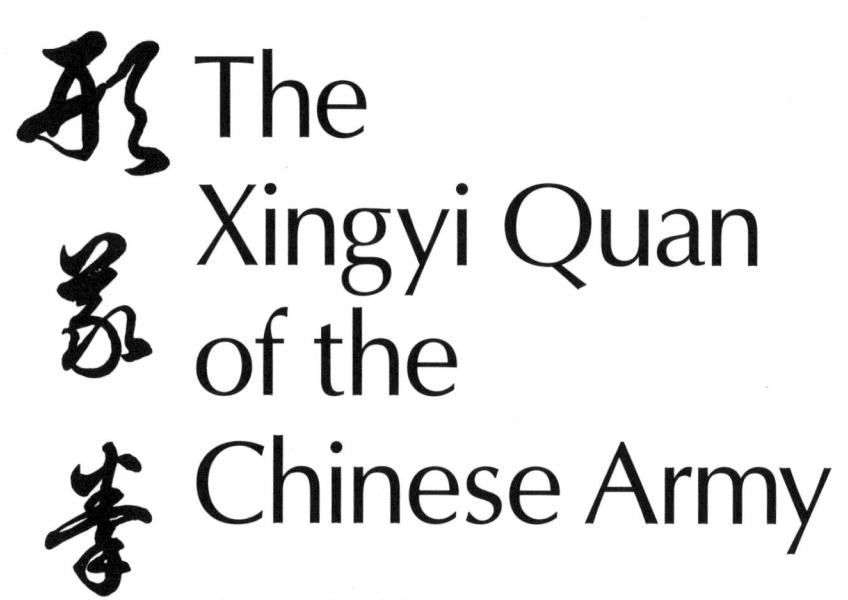

Huang Bo Nien's
*Xingyi Fist and Weapon Instruction*

## Dennis Rovere
with translation by Chow Hon Huen

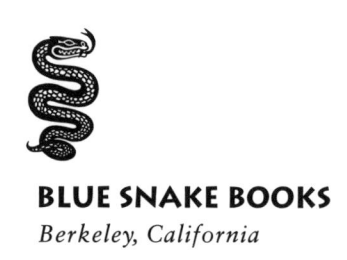

**BLUE SNAKE BOOKS**
*Berkeley, California*

Copyright © 2008 by Dennis Rovere. All rights reserved. No portion of this book, except for brief review, may be reproduced, stored in a retrieval system, or transmitted in any form or by any means—electronic, mechanical, photocopying, recording, or otherwise—without written permission of the publisher. For information contact Blue Snake Books c/o North Atlantic Books.

Published by Blue Snake Books

Blue Snake Books' publications are distributed by
North Atlantic Books
P.O. Box 12327
Berkeley, California 94712

Cover and book design by Brad Greene
Printed in the United States of America

*The Xingyi Quan of the Chinese Army: Huang Bo Nien's "Xingyi Fist and Weapon Instruction"* is sponsored by the Society for the Study of Native Arts and Sciences, a nonprofit educational corporation whose goals are to develop an educational and cross-cultural perspective linking various scientific, social, and artistic fields; to nurture a holistic view of arts, sciences, humanities, and healing; and to publish and distribute literature on the relationship of mind, body, and nature.

North Atlantic Books' publications are available through most bookstores. For further information, call 800-733-3000 or visit our websites at www.northatlanticbooks.com and www.bluesnakebooks.com.

Library of Congress Cataloging-in-Publication Data

Rovere, Dennis, 1952-
  The xingyi quan of the Chinese army: Huang Bo Nien's Xingyi fist and weapon instruction / by Dennis Rovere; with translation by Chow Hon Huen.
       p. cm.
  Chinese uniform title not available.
  Summary: "Presents an in-depth explanation of the original text of an important martial arts manual, including a look at the actual combat applications of xingyi as taught to the Chinese army"—Provided by publisher.
  ISBN 978-1-58394-257-4
  1. Hand to hand fighting, Oriental. 2. Martial arts—China. I. Title.
  GV1112.R68 2008
  796.815—dc22
                                                                    2008026133
                                                                    CIP

1 2 3 4 5 6 7 8 9 UNITED 14 13 12 11 10 09 08

— **Dedication** —

To my teacher,
COLONEL CHANG HSIANG WU,
former chief instructor of military strategy and xingyi
at the Central Military Academy
(Chong Yang Jun Shiao)
at Nanjing.

# ACKNOWLEDGMENTS

We would like to thank the following people for their support in this project:

**Lindsey Brady,** senior student and good friend. We especially want to thank him for his work as an outstanding attacker in all of our books and training DVDs.

**Abraham Dueck** for his patience in taking the photographs ("just one more, Abe") in Chapters 2 and 4.

**J. Richard Strang** for the photographs in Chapter 3 and his willingness to film in −5°C weather.

**Brian Kennedy** and **Elizabeth Guo** for their friendship, kindness, and willingness to go out of their way to help us.

**Jess O'Brien** for encouragement and for "pitching" this book to the publisher.

**Erin Wiegand** at North Atlantic Books for making the whole publishing process painless.

# SPECIAL ACKNOWLEDGMENT

When translating this book, I was overcome with sadness for the Chinese people during the early years of the Republic. The fact that our country was occupied by foreign governments and was later under attack reminded me of the countries currently at war, and this also saddens me.

Throughout China, many good men recognized the problems facing the country at that time. They used their knowledge and their hearts to try and make a difference for their country—and they did! They were leaders because they not only changed the old, conservative attitudes of martial artists but also gave hope to the military and the people as a whole. As a result of their dedication, there came about a significant change in the military history of China. Today both Taiwan and Mainland China have strong and well-trained military forces, and martial arts are always emphasized. Because of this, I think these good men deserve our respect.

Chow Hon Huen

PLEASE NOTE: The creators and publishers of this book are not and will not be responsible, in any way whatsoever, for any improper use made by anyone of the information contained in this book. All use of the aforementioned information must be made in accordance with what is permitted by law, and any damage liable to be caused as a result thereof will be the exclusive responsibility of the user. In addition, he or she must adhere strictly to the safety rules contained in the book, both in training and in actual implementation of the information presented herein. This book is intended for use in conjunction with ongoing lessons and personal training with an authorized expert. It is not a substitute for formal training. It is the sole responsibility of every person planning to train in the techniques described in this book to consult a licensed physician in order to obtain complete medical information on his or her personal ability and limitations. The instructions and advice printed in this book are not in any way intended as a substitute for medical, mental, or emotional counseling with a licensed physician or health-care provider.

# CONTENTS

| | |
|---|---|
| Foreword by Dr. Paul Chao | xv |
| Preface by the Translators | xvii |
|     *The Original Text* | xviii |
|     *Notes on This Translation* | xix |
| First Foreword to the Chinese Edition | xxi |
| Second Foreword to the Chinese Edition | xxiii |
| Third Foreword to the Chinese Edition | xxiv |
| Fourth Foreword to the Chinese Edition | xxv |
| Objective of the Book by Huang Bo Nian | xxvii |
| Preface by Huang Bo Nian | xxix |

## Chapter 1     1

| | |
|---|---|
| Section I: Explanation of the Five Element Theory | 1 |
| Background of the Five Element Theory | 3 |
| Section II: The Five Fists | 3 |
| Section III: The Linking Fist Form | 4 |
| Section IV: The Four Tips (Ends or Extremities) | 5 |
| Section V: The Eight Rules or Secrets | 6 |
| Section VI: The Nine Songs of the Beginning Position | 8 |

## Chapter 2 — 13

| | |
|---|---|
| Xingyi in the Chinese Army | 13 |
| Section I: Standing Position | 15 |
| Section II: Right Half Turn Position | 16 |
| Section III: Opening Position | 16 |
| Explanation of the Half Turn and Opening Positions | 17 |
| Section IV: Splitting Fist Route Illustration | 21 |
| Section V: Illustration of Splitting Fist | 22 |
| First Application of Action #2 | 24 |
| Second Application of Action #2 | 25 |
| Action #3: Counterattack Using the Landing Position | 26 |
| Application of the Neck Break | 26 |
| Section VI: Turning Around in Splitting Fist | 27 |
| Section VII: Drilling Fist Foot Pattern | 27 |
| Section VIII: Illustration of Drilling Fist | 28 |
| Applications of Drilling Fist | 30 |
| Section IX: Turning Around in Drilling Fist | 33 |
| Section X: Crushing Fist | 33 |
| Section XI: Turning Around in Crushing Fist | 34 |
| Increasing Mechanical Efficiency | 35 |
| Action #3: Moving from Action #2 into the Turning Position | 36 |
| Applications of Action #3 | 38 |
| Section XII: Pounding Fist | 40 |
| Section XIII: Illustration of Pounding Fist | 41 |
| Application Against an Empty Hand Attack | 42 |
| Application Against a Knife Attack | 43 |

| | |
|---|---|
| Section XIV: Turning Around in Pounding Fist | 44 |
| Section XV: Crossing Fist | 44 |
| Section XVI: Actions of Crossing Fist | 45 |
| Section XVII: Turning Around in Crossing Fist | 47 |
| Section XVIII: Explanation of Linking Fist's Opening and Stepping Diagram | 47 |
| Section XIX: Illustration of Linking Fist | 48 |
| Section XX: Turning Around in Linking Fist | 54 |
| Pici Training | 55 |

# Chapter 3 — 61

| | |
|---|---|
| Section I: Rifle and Bayonet Training | 61 |
| Holding Rifle and Standing at Attention | 62 |
| Ready Position | 62 |
| Explanation of Thrusting | 64 |
| Thrusting I | 68 |
| Explanation of Body Alignment | 69 |
| Drills for Thrusting I | 69 |
| Thrusting II | 76 |
| Drills for Thrusting II | 77 |
| Applications of Thrusting I and Thrusting II | 79 |
| Joint Attacks | 81 |
| Thrusting III | 81 |
| Drills for Thrusting III | 83 |
| Applications of Thrusting III | 85 |
| Thrusting IV | 87 |

| | |
|---|---|
| Explanation of Thrusting IV | 88 |
| Applications of Thrusting IV | 89 |
| More Actions of Thrusting IV | 92 |
| Ten Continuous Flowing Actions | 94 |
| Turning Around to Face Opponent | 98 |
| Explanation of Ten Continuous Flowing Actions | 98 |

# Chapter 4   103

| | |
|---|---|
| Common Misconceptions Regarding the Xingyi Military Sabre | 103 |
| Important Fundamentals for Handling the Two-Handed Sabre | 105 |
| Section I: Holding Sabre Method (Form) | 105 |
| Section II: Chopping Sabre Method | 106 |
| Explanation of Raising Sabre Pose | 108 |
| Application of Chopping Sabre Method | 110 |
| Action #2: Right Position | 114 |
| Explanation of Action #2: Consecutive Downward Slashes | 115 |
| Action #3: Turning Around | 116 |
| Application of Action #3 | 118 |
| Section III: Drilling Sabre Method | 119 |
| Explanation of Circular Movement | 121 |
| Application of Action #1 | 122 |
| Action #2: Right Position | 123 |
| Action #3 | 124 |
| Section IV: Crushing Sabre Method | 125 |
| Application of Action #1 | 126 |
| Action #2 | 127 |

| | |
|---|---|
| Action #3 | 128 |
| Section V: Pounding Sabre Method | 129 |
| First Application of Action #1 (Close-Range Attack) | 130 |
| Second Application of Action #1 (Long-Range Attack) | 131 |
| Action #2 | 132 |
| Application of Action #2 | 133 |
| Action#3 | 134 |
| Section VI: Crossing Sabre Form | 135 |
| Application of Action#1 | 137 |
| Action #2 | 138 |
| Action #3 | 139 |
| | |
| Xingyi Terms in English and Chinese | 140 |
| Xingyi Lineage of Dennis Rovere | 143 |
| About the Authors | 144 |

# FOREWORD

Throughout China's history, vast numbers of books have been written on every aspect of human life. Unfortunately, only a small percentage of them have been translated into Western languages. Because of this, many misconceptions regarding Chinese culture are promulgated in the West, both wittingly and unwittingly. Even the most superficial of readings of Chinese literature would dispel these fictions, but the language barrier has blocked the Western reader.

In no field is this sad state of affairs more apparent than in the history of Chinese martial arts. I have three reasons to be delighted in recommending this book to students of Chinese martial arts in the West:

- *Xingyi Fist and Weapon Instruction* by Huang Bo Nian is one of the classic texts of *xingyi quan*. It outlines in a straightforward, no-nonsense way the techniques and applications necessary for victory in battle. (Chinese martial arts are, after all, the development of fighting skill and the character required to integrate that skill into a moral, productive life.)
- Chow Hon Huen has faithfully rendered the original Chinese text into modern English, thereby bringing the ideas clearly forth.
- Mr. Rovere's teacher, Colonel Chang Hsiang Wu (an acknowledged xingyi master himself), and Huang were contemporaries. As well, the Government of the Republic of China has recognized Mr. Rovere's accomplishments as a disciple of Col. Chang. It is his understanding that transforms this book from an academic exercise to a document from which the serious student can actually learn.

I trust you will find this book enlightening and I wish you the best in your further studies of Chinese culture.

—Paul Chao, MA, EdD
Cultural Attaché Emeritus, Government of the Republic of China

# PREFACE
## BY THE TRANSLATORS

This book began in 1988 from a discussion with my teacher, Colonel Chang Hsiang Wu. I was interested in writing a practical book on xingyi with emphasis on how it was taught and used in the Chinese army during the Chinese-Japanese war.

In the 1930s, Colonel Chang had been military strategy and xingyi instructor at the *Chung Yan Jun Shiao, Nanjing*—the Central Military Academy at Nanjing. He began his xingyi training in 1915 and either trained with, or was acquainted with, most of the xingyi masters at the time, including this book's author, Huang Bo Nian. One of Colonel Chang's responsibilities at the military academy was to train officer-instructors in the fundamentals of xingyi as a modern military close-combat art.

When I proposed my project to Colonel Chang, he immediately suggested I present a two-part series. The first part would consist of a translation of Huang Bo Nian's book *Xingyi Fist and Weapon Instruction*. The second part would

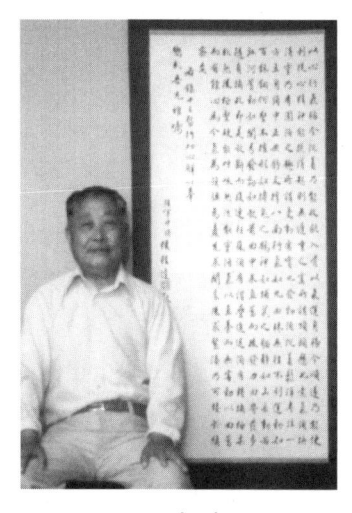

Col. Chang Hsiang Wu, 1906–1997.

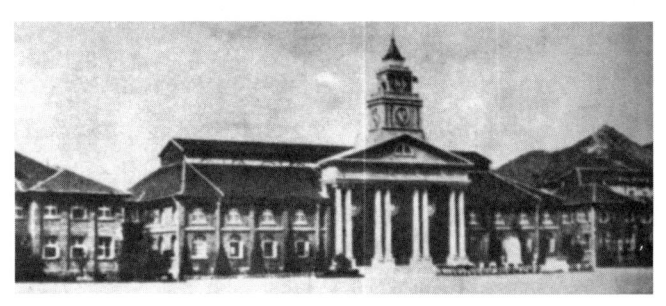

Central Military Academy, Nanjing.

show applications, theory, and training format as practiced at the military academy.

## THE ORIGINAL TEXT

Written in 1928, *Xingyi Fist and Weapon Instruction* is a book of historical significance. It was the first attempt to systematically adapt a traditional Chinese martial art for use in modern warfare. The book was presented as a means of progressive training, from empty hand to combat with weapons. It formed the basis of empty hand weapons training both at the Central Military Academy and elsewhere.

The drawback to Huang's book is that it is written more as a drill instructor's manual than a "do-it-yourself" guide. The assumption was that the person using the manual already knew xingyi. As a result, empty hand applications are not discussed. When applications are described, as in the rifle-bayonet and sabre sections, they are done so only in reference to the single-person drills.

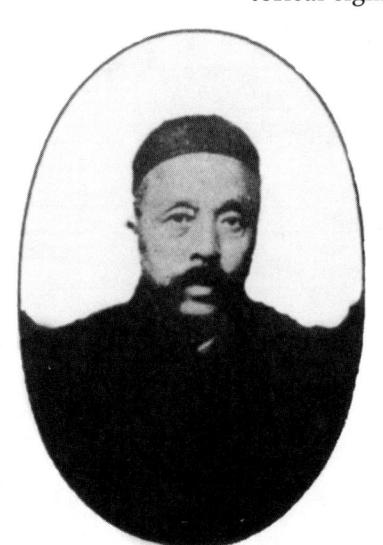

Huang Bo Nian, 1880–1954.

Huang was not the first, nor the only, instructor to propose using the techniques of xingyi as a method of teaching close combat to the army. The famous xingyi master Sun Lu Tang taught for the government in Beijing between 1919 and 1924 and was commissioned as a lieutenant in the army in approximately 1920. Additionally, Wang Yu Shen (also known as Wang Xiang Zhai, c. 1890–1963), the founder of *yi quan,* trained military personnel.

Huang was not just a theorist. In 1931, he was hired to teach his method for sabre, bayonet, and empty hand at the Nanjing Zhong Yang Guo Shu Guan (Central National Arts/Martial Arts Academy, Nanjing).

By 1934 the men at the Martial Arts Academy spent 2½ hours per week training rifle and bayonet techniques and 3 hours per week in empty hand xingyi practice. With the establishment of the Central Military Academy at Nanjing prior to this time period and the impending all-out conflict with Japan, it is obvious that there was a serious need for Huang's methodology. In 1937, Huang took a position as a martial arts instructor at the Zhong Jing Military Academy.

In addition to famous teachers, the success of xingyi stylists in the national martial arts competition held in Nanjing in 1928 may have contributed to its popularity within certain units of the Chinese army.

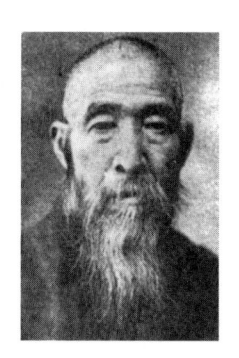

Sun Lu Tang, 1861–1933.

## NOTES ON THIS TRANSLATION

In preparing the translated portion of this book, Chow Hon Huen, who did the direct translation, and I have chosen to make the following compromises:

- Superfluous text has been eliminated or clarified. Chinese authors tend to repeat phrases for emphasis. Additionally, the convoluted and confusing blend of classical and modern Chinese as well as the hidden meanings makes a literal English translation confusing to read. We have chosen, for the sake of brevity and to avoid ambiguity, not to directly follow Huang's sometimes-repetitious writing style.
- Directions in the Chinese text have been presented in the passive voice. Since the second person in English ("you") and the present tense read better and make a clearer, more direct connection with instructions and orders, we have chosen to follow this format throughout.
- In some places in the text we have chosen to follow "mood and flow" rather than a literal translation. This is not to say we have altered the text. On the contrary, for important places where a discrepancy would exist or where we have chosen to leave the original Chinese word in place, an explanatory comment in parentheses and italics has been provided. Literal translations of some words have been enclosed in square brackets and show an alternate or more direct

(and often confusing) translation of the word or phrase. We have tried to keep this to a minimum, but because of the nature of Huang's text, it was sometimes unavoidable.

Although often quoted, original copies of this book are actually quite rare. For the copies that do exist, the photos in these books are less than perfect. Additionally, the author used a "ghosting" technique consisting of the dotted outline of the demonstrator superimposed on the photograph. This method actually causes the photos to be even less legible, as the dots tend to blend into the background with some printing methods.

Because of the historical value of Huang's work, we have included all the original photographs (such as they are) from the best copies that were available to us. We have also reposed these sequences and labeled them with the letter "m" and where applicable with a number, to make the information clearer to our readers.

We have included a cross-section of applications described, but not illustrated, in the original. Sequences of moves in the applications have been designated with a figure number followed by a lowercase letter of the alphabet (a, b, c, and so on).

While there are discrepancies between Huang's explanation and the method taught at the Central Military Academy at the time, they are, for the most part, minor. Where variations are presented, they are done so as an adjunct and have been noted as such.

—Dennis Rovere
—Chow Hon Huen

# FIRST FOREWORD
## TO THE CHINESE EDITION

When Confucius spoke about the superiority of man, there was a difference between North and South. (The suspicion is that Southerners are better in literature.) During the Kingdom of Yin, there were many sad scholars. Because of the geographic barriers, people did not realize that this is a man-made phenomenon. Ever since the Shang Wu Jen De Hui *(Martial Arts and Morals Association)* was established, the number of people coming *(to train)* every year and the number of people who have finished has changed the general concept of society.

Last year the Nationalist Government established and eagerly sponsored training facilities to promote martial arts. In addition, Mr. Zhang Zi Min and Li Feng Chen went around and enthusiastically promoted martial arts—so much so that it has become a trend. People from the North came to observe. Scholars from the South also expressed the same interest. Now that we have both Northern and Southern interest, we are not speaking about a change in one or two people but rather a *(national)* trend.

The Shang Wu Jen De Hui is going to publish a series of martial arts and specialty books to promote martial arts. From now on, people will be able to understand the source and methods of these secret, ancient martial arts styles. Everyone in the country can share and understand their origins. I hope the association members "keep up the good work."

Morality in martial arts is for transforming all heroes into righteous persons. Because of this, the people of our country will become persons with wisdom and bravery and we will not have to worry about insults or suppression by other people. Since Japanese *bushido* originated in our country, we must now restart its promotion *(among ourselves)*. This change is a way for our nation to regain pride in itself. I am pleased to write this foreword.

    Seventeenth year of the Republic, October
    —Wang Zheng Ting

# SECOND FOREWORD
## TO THE CHINESE EDITION

To learn, you must focus instead of trying to absorb too many "bits and pieces." When you focus, it is easy to excel. If you learn only bits and pieces, it will be difficult to attain success. The study of martial arts is the same.

Our country has many different styles of martial arts. If you do not learn correctly, the quality will deteriorate. Mr. Huang Bo Nian understands this theory and has used his knowledge and time to write this fist and weapon instructional manual. He uses the five element fists in xingyi quan to open the door and allow students to learn progressively and avoid the problem of learning bits and pieces. He also follows the original style when he talks about weapons.

This book is an instructional manual and who would disagree? *(This is a compliment, referring to Huang's high degree of accomplishment and sincerity in presenting "real" xingyi to the public.)*

I believe that the publication of this book will benefit future generations of students. They will understand our way. This is why I am most happy to write this foreword.

Seventeenth year *(of the Republic)*, December 4th
—Sun Lu Tang, Shanghai

# THIRD FOREWORD
## TO THE CHINESE EDITION

Society is composed of different individuals. Countries are composed of different societies. This is why you must look at a country's people if you want to see its strength. The military is a special society. It is composed of many individuals who must suppress riots and defend the country. They have great responsibilities. If they are called a strong army, it is for many reasons—the first being the physique *(physical prowess)* of its soldiers.

Mr. Huang Bo Nian, the author, showed me his books on fist and bayonet forms. The first book is written by his teacher Li Cun Yi. The second book is written by Mr. Huang himself. I read both and noted his movements use strategy and speed and display a high level of skill. One action becomes many movements. Many movements revert to one action. The changes are endless and practical. He reedited the book and added diagrams and commands so it would be easy to teach and learn. He combined his two books into one, called it a fist and weapon instructional manual, and had it published. The public can follow the instructions and diagrams to practice and strengthen our country. So this *(manual)* is not just for the soldiers' benefit.

—Huang Zhen Kui

# FOURTH FOREWORD
## TO THE CHINESE EDITION

A country's strength or weakness lies with its people. Strength or weakness of its people lies in their physical prowess. This determines winning or losing, surviving or perishing. This is why martial arts must be revitalized.

I did not complete my *(school or formal)* education. Instead I took up the study of martial arts. In the late Qing Dynasty, I started to learn xingyi and *bagua zhang* from Mr. Zhang Zhao Dong. Later I received more instruction from Mr. Li Cun Yi.

This year, Mr. Zhang Zhi Jiang and Mr. Li Fang Chen established a martial arts school. Many people now follow them. My colleagues and I formed the Shang Wu Jen De Hui. It took three months to organize. We are also looking to publish our books in order to spread knowledge. My friend Mr. Huang Jie Zi *(another name for Huang Bo Nian)* is the senior student of Mr. Li Cun Yi. He is also one of the directors of our association.

This book is primarily designed as a fist and weapon instruction manual. He uses the five element fist and linking form of xingyi quan as its basis [basic level]. He uses bayonet and sword as a means of progressing to the advanced stage. He uses commands as an instructional method. This is particularly suitable for military schools. With the route illustrations, the book is presented in an orderly and clear manner. This is an outstanding and new approach in martial art circles. This is our first publication. I also posed for the photographs and wrote this foreword. I hope it will be published soon to present it to the "good men of our country" to read.

—Jiang Rong Qiao
Seventeenth year *(of the Republic)*, December 4th

# OBJECTIVE OF THE BOOK
## BY HUANG BO NIAN

*(In the original Chinese text, this section was placed at the beginning of the book. Since this could be confusing to the reader, we thought it was better situated immediately before the Preface.)*

The objective is to combine the three categories—five elements and linking method; stab and thrust *(bayonet)* techniques; and chopping *(sabre)* methods—into one book. Diagrams and route patterns *(stepping diagrams)* are included to make it easier for the practitioner to learn.

**Empty Hand Practice:** You need to memorize the Songs *(see below)*. Only then can you practice correct methods for training your body. This way *(of learning)* is better than the methods followed by people who did not start from the basics and only learn bits and pieces.

**Bayonet Practice:** All of the bayonet methods derive from famous ancient and current spear experts. These techniques all come from years of practice, teaching, and practical combat experience. If you practice with the bayonet, you will increase your efficiency.

**Sabre Practice:** Sabre methods in this book take as their basis the *five element sword method*. In order to have sufficient strength in the wrist, both hands are required to use the sabre.

Each movement is simple and practical. All are easy to learn, and are better than fancy techniques that are only good to look at.

After practicing the *five element empty hand method*, you can start learning thrusting and chopping techniques. Movements involving chopping with the sabre are based directly upon the five element empty hands. Thrusting with the spear requires familiarity with empty hand methods. If not, you will only know how to use force from the wrist. You will not understand how to use force that springs from the ground. Thrusting is ferocious. You cannot learn it before you finish the five element empty hand method.

For *continuous thrusting*, the steps are the same as for *empty hand linking form*. This is why you must learn the empty hand linking form before you learn the linking and thrusting form.

This style does not require strain [degree of difficulty] such as bending knees and breaking waist. Nor does it require the exertion involved in high jumping. Even older people can practice this. The author thinks that these techniques are superior to other sword methods.

This book took several months to finish. The author would like to thank Liu Guang Yu, Ge Yi, and Wang Guo Jie, who did the diagrams.

—Huang Bo Nian

*(The "Songs" are short rhyming phrases that emphasize important points in training. Each line contains a set number of characters. The number of characters is left to the discretion of the writer. In Huang's book, for example, there are four words per line. The reason they are called "Songs" is to differentiate them from poetry, which has strict rules of composition.)*

# PREFACE
## BY HUANG BO NIAN

The way of martial arts has a long history. In prehistoric times, men and animals competed for survival. Strength was the main factor. Intelligence was secondary. Later man competed with man with both intelligence and strength. This was the beginning of martial arts. This is why a great deal of literature is devoted to the study of strategy and why physical conflict is recorded in history books. Many books discuss the techniques of hand-to-hand combat and swords *(weapons)*. It is rumored that Yueh Fei's xingyi fist book (a secret text) was developed by Da Mo while he was staying at Song Shan [Song Mountain]. He developed this system for conditioning the body. Even though one cannot clearly determine its origin, there is a possibility they are connected in some way.

In one Western country, the people admire martial prowess. In general, the people glorify bloodshed and despise the shedding of tears. People there not only have a high level of physical fitness; they also have the skills to fight ferocious animals.

In ancient times in our country, weapons were the main means of attack and defense. All martial artists had their own specialties. For example, there is Jiang Mo's sabre, Yueh Fei's spear, and the sword of Hon Yeuh. They were all famous at one time in history.

Unfortunately, the fist forms in our country were kept a secret. They were always taught orally and never recorded in written form. This is why many excellent fist forms were lost. In later generations, students who wanted to learn regretted the missed opportunities. Although there are a few people who did study, they were only able to learn 20 to 30 percent. How can you reach the top of a mountain *(a high level of skill)* and be as good as the ancestors? This is due to the ancestors' stubbornness, fears, lack of trust, and suspicions. This is the biggest obstacle in the martial arts world.

During the Southern Tang and early Qing Dynasties, finally some books were written on the fist forms. These books helped students find a path for learning. It is unfortunate that in the late Qing Dynasty we became westernized. We recognized *(adopted)* firearms and our military systems changed. Our country absorbed other people's shallowness and forgot our own country's essence. The standard of martial arts deteriorated. This is so sad.

We have to understand that the strength of an army depends upon the bravery of the soldiers. If the soldiers are weak they still could not proficiently use sophisticated firearms. If soldiers are brave [fit and trained], even though they are empty handed or engage in close combat, they still have a chance to win. This is why proper training is the most urgent priority in the military. To train good soldiers, we must promote martial arts. *(If we do this)* all civilians will have a desire to learn martial arts and this will give us a perfect army. Presently, our firearms and aircraft are improving. However, the best means to fight our enemy is still through combat troops. This is why we all think martial arts are the most important training in our army.

There are currently many books. Unfortunately, some of the context is outdated and not suitable for the present times. Some of the words are too hard to understand; this makes learning difficult. Because it is not very clear, it is hard to teach this subject to the public. Because of this, I edited and updated Yueh Fei's fist form book that was given to me by my teacher Mr. Li Cun Yi. I used battlefield experience to change this book into a fist and weapon instruction manual. I also added illustrations and detailed explanations. I used military commands for the movements. I used modern Chinese instead of ancient Chinese to make it easier for students to learn. Those who teach can use this book to teach progressively and can receive good results when instructing the public.

These are the thoughts I have after studying martial arts. I am sure this will be supported by people who share the same interest. Compared to the unlimited variations of martial arts, one person's wisdom is limited.

I believe there are imperfections in this book. I wish people who have this same interest will please teach me. *(This is a humble way of saying "I would appreciate it if you read my book and give me your honest comments.")*

Seventeenth year *(of the Republic)*, October
—Huang Bo Nian

# Chapter 1

## SECTION I: EXPLANATION OF THE FIVE ELEMENT THEORY

The five elements are Metal, Wood, Water, Fire, and Earth. In the body, these elements are matched with five internal organs and five external features. These organs and their elemental counterparts are:

Heart belongs to Fire

Spleen belongs to Earth

Liver belongs to Wood

Lungs belong to Metal

Kidneys belong to Water

This relationship is referred to as the *five elements placed internally*. Additionally, external features correspond to the internal organs:

Eyes connect to liver

Nose connects to lungs

Tongue connects to heart

Ears connect to kidneys

Base of nose connects to spleen

This linking is often referred to as *five elements placed externally*.

The five elements have an *assisting theory* and a *hindering theory*. The assisting relationships of the elements are:

Metal assists Water

Water assists Wood

Wood assists Fire

Fire assists Earth

Earth assists Metal

The hindering relationships among the elements are:

Metal hinders Wood

Wood hinders Earth

Earth hinders Water

Water hinders Fire

Fire hinders Metal

These groups are all diverse and expansive. *(This means that the five element theory is applicable to a large number of phenomena, not just the ones mentioned here.)*

Scholars of the Han Dynasty used the five element theory to explain much of the phenomena occurring in nature. After the Han Dynasty, people stopped believing in the elemental relationships because they failed to see any real application for them. According to the author *(here Huang is referring to himself)*, the theories of assisting and hindering are not inappropriate—that is why the fist forms are named for the elements. Understanding and applying the theory of assisting and hindering helps to strengthen both internal and external power. In everyday practice, assisting theory is used to improve health and increase power. When preparing to fight the enemy, hindering theory is used.

## BACKGROUND OF THE FIVE ELEMENT THEORY

Mentioned in the *Book of History, Mo Tzu,* and other writings, the five element theory *(wu xing)* is more appropriately known as the five agents, actions, or operations.

Like its counterpart yin and yang, the five element theory was an early attempt to discuss metaphysics and cosmology. Unlike yin and yang, the five element theory was cyclical in nature. The elements do not refer to physical substances but rather to metaphysical forces.

In Han times, the analogies created by these agents were extremely complex and encompassed a large number of subjects. They were applied to such diverse things as virtues, colors, smells, sacrifices, rulers and dynasties, parts of the body, seasons, and the "ten heavenly stems" and "twelve earthly branches."

There is no indication in any of my research that the five fists of xingyi were developed from this theory. It is more likely that the five element theory was overlaid on top of the fists to provide a rudimentary means of systematizing and teaching combat strategy and applications.

## SECTION II: EXPLANATION OF THE FIVE FISTS

Crushing *(beng)*, drilling *(zuan)*, splitting *(pi)*, pounding [exploding] *(pao)*, and crossing [horizontal] *(heng)* are the names of the five fist *(wu quan)* forms.

> In crushing, the fist is shaped like an arrow and therefore belongs to Wood.
>
> In drilling, the fist is shaped like lightning and therefore belongs to Water.

In splitting, the fist is shaped like an axe and therefore belongs to Metal.

In pounding, the fist is cannon shaped and therefore belongs to Fire.

In crossing, the fist is shaped like a spring and therefore belongs to Earth.

Using assisting theory we observe that:

Crushing fist assists pounding fist

Drilling fist assists crushing fist

Splitting fist assists drilling fist

Pounding fist assists crossing fist

Crossing fist assists splitting fist

Because everything is born from Earth, crossing fist is capable of assisting every other fist.

From the hindering theory we note that:

Crushing fist hinders crossing fist

Drilling fist hinders pounding fist

Splitting fist hinders crushing fist

Pounding fist hinders splitting fist

Crossing fist hinders drilling fist

# SECTION III: THE LINKING FIST FORM

The five element linking fist form [five element fist combination form] connects the individual fist forms into a group. Although movement in the linking form is cyclical *(attacking and withdrawing)*, unexpected changes occur all the time—changes that have many subtleties hidden within them. Originally this form was named *forward, backward, linking fist form* [forward, backward, continuous fist form]. Now this form is simply called linking fist form [continuous fist form].

The continuous fist form is based upon the individual five element fist forms. It is therefore considered the advanced form while the individual forms are considered basic forms. This advanced form is divided into ten sections, half of which are forward *(offensive)* while the other half are backward *(defensive)*. As there are relatively few moves in this style, the linking form has been extended to allow for greater continuity *(i.e., fewer pauses between repetitions)*. To extend the form, do not turn around until crushing fist *(is performed)*. Continue with the second sequence. Repeat this until forty sets have been completed.

All fist forms are for practical use. Linking fist connects the five element fist forms. Depending on the situation, you can either use fist [hand closed] or palm [palm extended, hand open]. Here, linking fist becomes linking palm. Although changing from palm to fist *(and vice versa)* is for empty hand use, it can be directly applied to weapons. No matter what the weapon is—spear, knife, sword or staff—all can be used for thrusting, chopping, and slashing. These motions are simple extensions of empty hand techniques.

## SECTION IV: THE FOUR TIPS (ENDS OR EXTREMITIES)

Tips or ends of the blood, flesh, tendons, or bones are called *dou*. Hair is the tip of the blood, tongue is the tip of the flesh, fingers are the tips of our tendons [sinews], and teeth are the tips of the bones. If one tenses all these extremities, it results in a change in one's usual appearance. Such a change can be used to startle or frighten others.

**Blood tip.** When one has angry *Qi (air; energy)* filling the chest, blood circulates and the hair stands on end. When this occurs, the enemy will be frightened. Although hairs are tiny, it is not difficult to use them to defeat [destroy the courage of] your opponent.

**Flesh tip.** When you roll your tongue, your Qi sinks. Even though one is confronted by a mountain, it can be knocked down. Flesh becomes hard as iron and spirit is brave. The power of the tongue makes the enemy lose his courage [guts].

**Tendon tip.** Eagles and tigers are both ferocious [powerful]. This is because they use their claws *(fingers)* as weapons. They grab things with their hands and stomp them with their feet.

*"Wherever your claws are, you will succeed."*

**Bone tip.**

*"When one has courage, one is eager to fight."*

Bones tense up and teeth are shown. This gives the impression that one wants to chew the enemy's flesh. Veins show and the eyeballs bulge. This is the result of the teeth. It will make people terrified.

## SECTION V: THE EIGHT RULES OR SECRETS

In addition to the four tips are the eight rules or secrets. These are:

To be erect [top of the head is upright]

To hook

To circle

To be vicious

To hold

To let hang

To be bent

To be straight [upright]

When one is ready to open the stance, one will be prepared with these eight rules.

*"Conserve energy and grow Qi so your enemies will not control or overpower you. These are special characteristics of the five element fists."*

Each of these eight rules is subdivided into three types:

**Rule 1, to be erect.** Head is held erect and one looks up, not down. This is called *flying to the sky*. Hands push out and one has the *knocking down mountain power*. Tongue is held upward so that one has the *lion swallowing elephant position*. This is called the *three types to be erect*.

**Rule 2, to hook.** Shoulders hook so that strength will gather at the elbows. Palms hook so that the strength will be in your palm. Fingers hook so that the strength will be all over your body. This is called the *three types to hook*.

**Rule 3, to circle.** When the back is rounded, the strength will push your body forward. When the chest is rounded, both elbows will be full of power. When the *tiger mouth (curved space between thumb and index finger)* is rounded, then power can be sent out. This is called the *three types to circle*.

**Rule 4, to be vicious [poisonous].** The heart is as vicious as an angry fox that catches the rat. The eyes are as vicious as a hungry eagle watching the rabbit. The hands are as vicious as a hungry tiger grabbing a lamb. This is called the *three types to be vicious*.

**Rule 5, to hold.** One holds the Qi in the *dan tien*. This prevents Qi from escaping or spreading. Courage is held within the body. One does not lose his calm when facing danger. One uses the elbows to hold the upper body. If this is done, wherever one goes calm is not lost. This is called the *three types to hold*.

**Rule 6, to let hang** [drop or lower]. If Qi drops it will reach the dan tien. If shoulders drop they assist in pushing the elbows forward. If elbows drop the arms will be rounded. This is called the *three types to let hang*.

**Rule 7, to be bent** [not straight; curved; crooked]. Arms should be bent; if bent there is great power. The two hips should be bent; if bent strength will be full. Wrist should be bent; if bent there will be a great deal of strength. This is called the *three types to be bent*.

**Rule 8, to be straight** [upright]. If the neck is straight the Qi will reach the top of the head. If the waist is straight the strength will reach the four tips. If the knee is straight one is calm. This is called the *three types to be straight [upright]*.

## SECTION VI: THE NINE SONGS OF THE BEGINNING POSITION

**Body.** If one leans forward or backward, moves will not be powerful. If one leans left or right, body position is not correct. Straight but seems not straight. Not straight but seems straight. *(He can't determine your body position.)*

**Shoulders.** Head should be held upward while shoulders drop. Left shoulder bends while right shoulder follows the body. This allows strength to reach the hand.

**Arms.** Left arm extends to the right, front of the body, while right arm "plays" *(lightly rests)* on the ribs. It *(the arm)* looks straight but is actually not too straight. If arms are too curved one will be "unable to hit far" *(unable to reach the target)*. If arms are too straight there will not be enough power [force].

**Hands.** Right hand is held along the ribs. Left hand is level with the chest. Left hand drops slightly while right hand stretches with power. Both hands hold the position with the palms facing down. Strength [power] in each of the hands should be equal.

**Fingers.** All five fingers are slightly separated and take the shape of hooks. The tiger mouth is rounded so that the position looks both strong and soft. Power [strength] should reach the hands. Do not exert yourself.

**Hip** *(thigh)*. Left hip is in front while right hip supports the body at the back. The position should look straight but not too straight. It should look like a bow, but not exactly like a bow. Straight and curved positions should give the image of the *chicken [rooster] hip shape.*

**Feet.** Left foot points straight forward. If it points to the side the position is incorrect. Right foot points slightly to the side. Distance between heel of the front foot and toe of the rear foot is approximately 2 feet. All of the toes should grab the floor.

**Tongue.** The tongue is the tip of the flesh. If tongue is rolled the Qi will sink. If eyes are widened the dan tien will become stronger. If muscles are strong as iron the internal organs will also be strong.

**Buttocks.** If one lifts the buttocks the Qi reaches the four tips. If the two legs twist slightly the muscles in the buttocks tighten. If the position is too low the power will be lost. This is why it is better to be higher.

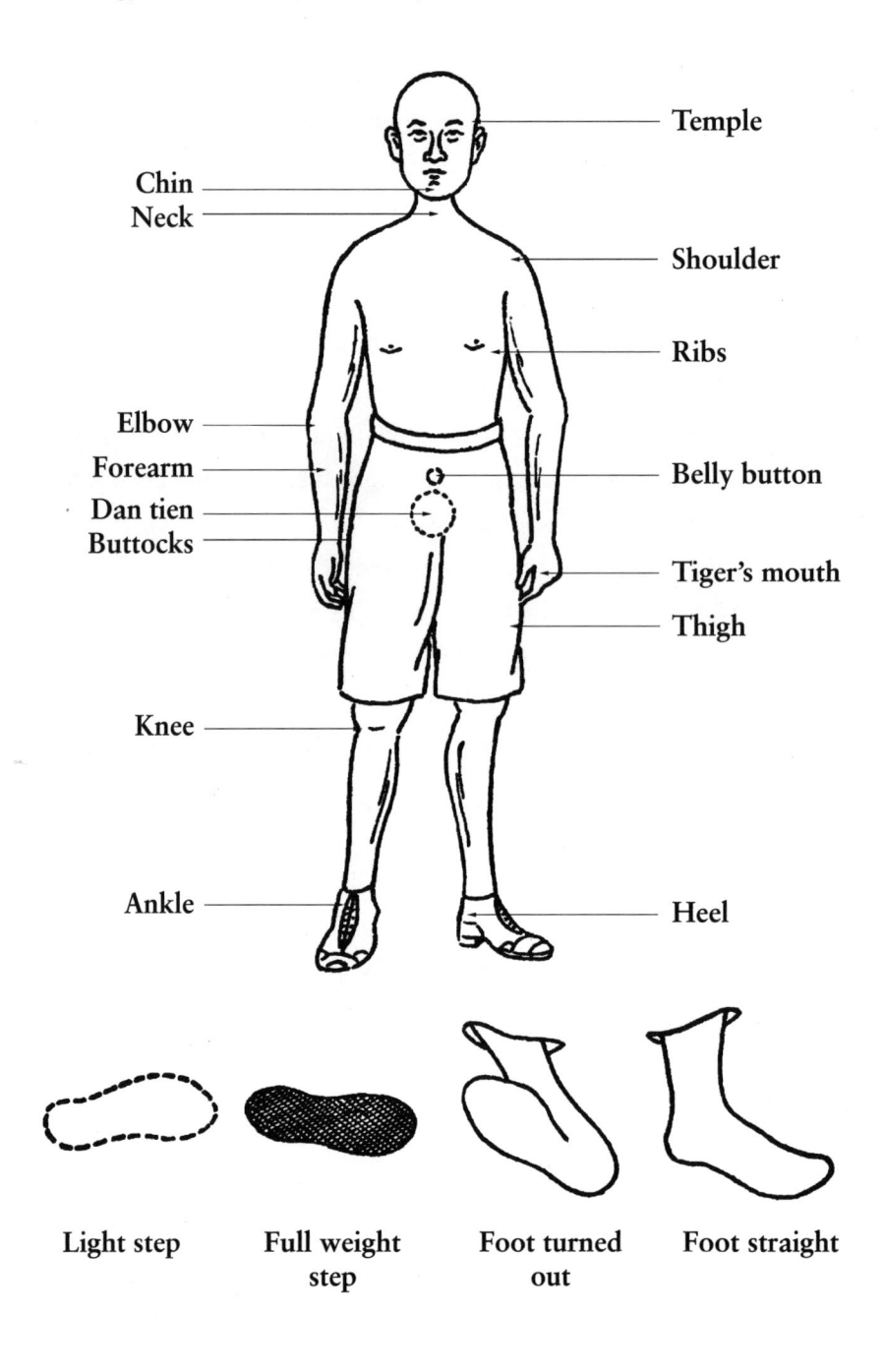

Temple
Chin
Neck
Shoulder
Ribs
Elbow
Forearm
Dan tien
Buttocks
Belly button
Tiger's mouth
Thigh
Knee
Ankle
Heel

Light step | Full weight step | Foot turned out | Foot straight

Figure 1-1.

| Weapon line | Turn (body) | Withdrawing | Advancing |

Yang palm

Standing fist

Yin palm

Upturned fist

Figure 1-2.

# Chapter 2

## XINGYI IN THE CHINESE ARMY

Because of limited time available for training, xingyi at the Central Military Academy placed emphasis primarily upon understanding the five fists, two-person and linking forms, and their practical applications—the same material contained in Huang's book. It was through a mastery of these basics that one is able to transform a single strike into a crippling blow. It is also from these fundamentals that all weapon applications evolve.

At the Central Military Academy, fist methods were taught in three stages over a period of one or two months. In order, these stages are:

Solo forms and basics

Applications and prearranged sparring

Free fighting

Although xingyi training was condensed, it nonetheless followed an orthodox method of instruction, with the fists taught as complete sequences. This allowed the officer to quickly develop a proper sense of timing, weight shifting, and stability—thereby accelerating his learning process.

## Attack Only

Another characteristic of military xingyi training was that initially no withdrawing or retreating movements are taught. This is important for several reasons:

It instilled in the soldier the idea of aggressive attack.

It taught the soldier to close distance and move inside an opponent's effective fighting range. This is of particular value when armed with a long weapon such as a rifle and bayonet.

## Continuous Flowing

In addition to forward movements only, all five element techniques utilize continuous flowing and alternating actions. This assists the practitioner in several ways:

Continuous flowing enables you to incorporate your body mass while delivering the blow. For example, in empty hand splitting fist, the momentum your body generates in the counterstrike is capable of breaking your opponent's neck.

In the sabre technique of splitting, the chopping and cutting actions of the sword are made more devastating by dropping the weight of the shoulders and arms. This results in a cut that penetrates all the way to the bone. Such a cut causes severe nerve and muscle damage as well as massive trauma or shock.

Continuous flowing teaches combatants to move easily and steadily over uneven terrain. Steps are kept low and reinforced so that there is no overextension. The twofold end result is an ability to change both level and angle of attack and an ability to deliver several crippling blows in quick succession.

Continuous flowing enables you to easily alternate actions so that both sides of the body are equally trained. Alternating sides when practicing is a fundamental characteristic of xingyi. This is true of empty hand training and particularly necessary in weapons application.

Over the years, however, I have noticed that many xingyi practitioners, especially those practicing sabre techniques, alternate their stepping but only block to one side of the body. As we will see both here and in Huang's descriptions of the applications in Chapter 3 and 4, both offensive and defensive moves are delivered to and from both sides of the body. To alternate stepping while only practicing blocking and cutting from one side of the body means you have only trained half the movements and are inadequately prepared for actual combat.

# SECTION I: STANDING POSITION

Stand with both feet side by side. Heels are together. Tips of your toes point outward at a 60-degree angle. Keep both legs straight but bend your knees slightly. Tuck in your abdomen. Push out your chest. Keep your shoulders level.

Arms hang comfortably *(by your sides)*. Turn palms slightly outward toward the front. Bend your hands a little and keep the five fingers together. Your little fingers should touch the center of your legs. Keep your head up, neck straight, and chin slightly lowered. Eyes are level. Look forward.

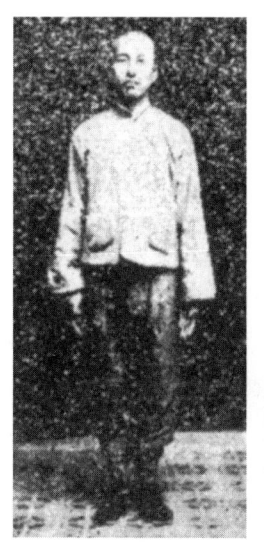

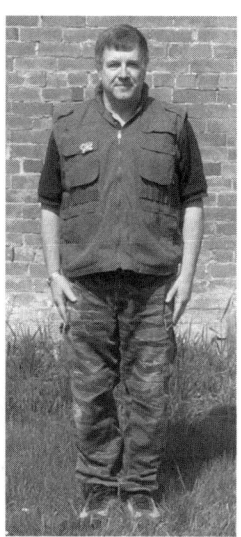

Figure 2-1.

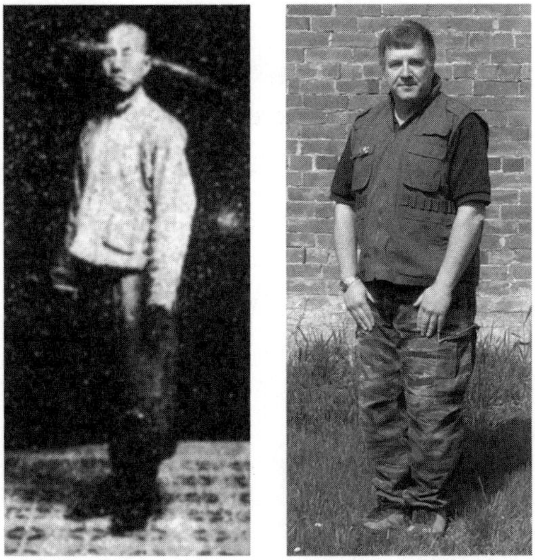

## SECTION II: RIGHT HALF TURN POSITION

To change from standing position to right half turn position, first slightly lift the tips of your feet. Next, use your heels as pivot points, and turn to the right. When the desired position is reached, set the tips of your feet down. Maintain the standing pose with both the arms and body. *Half face* your body to the right, but keep your head facing to the left *(front)*. Left foot points forward.

Figure 2-2.

## SECTION III: OPENING POSITION

The *opening position* (as shown in Figures 2-3, 2-3m1, and 2-3m2) is the starting position for both the five fists and all other forms. One should thoroughly understand the nine songs in order to make practice easier.

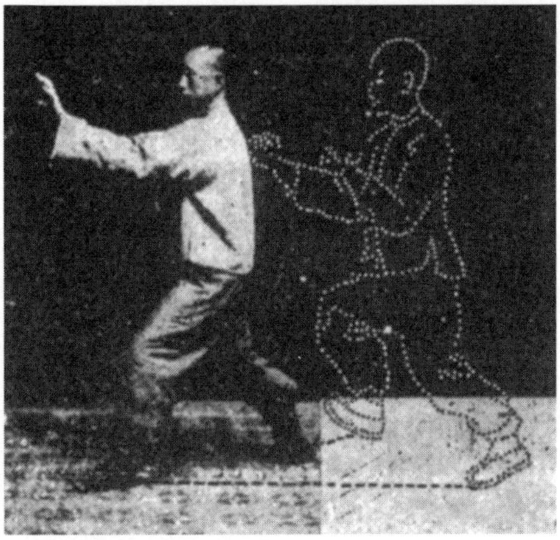

Figure 2-3.

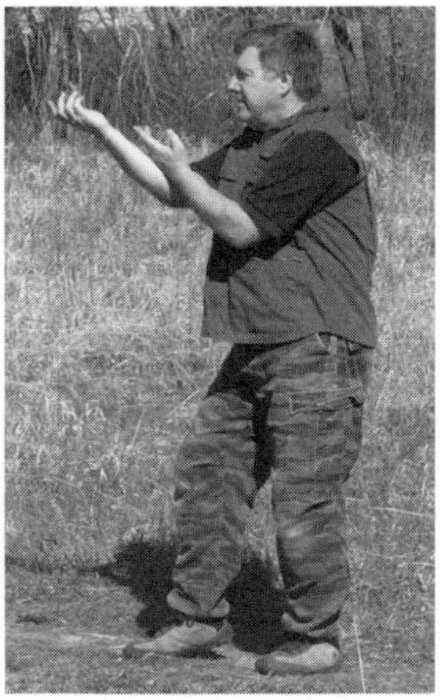

Figure 2-3m1.

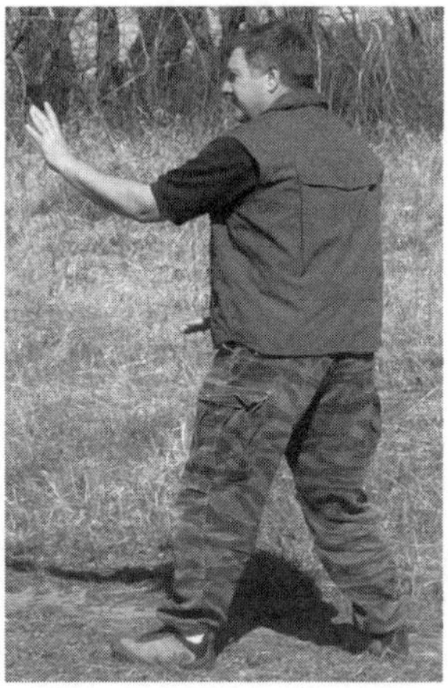

Figure 2-3m2.

# EXPLANATION OF THE HALF TURN AND OPENING POSITIONS

The half turn position is an important one and serves several purposes. The most obvious purpose is that it assists the arms in punching and striking. It is, in essence, the first link in the chain of energy transfer. From this position, the rear foot pushes against the ground. Because the ground resists, the force is sent back through the leg to the waist. As you turn back toward the front, using your hips and waist as a single unit, you allow this force to push out through the shoulder and arms to the fists, and ultimately into your target.

Your legs constitute approximately two-thirds of your body weight and are capable of generating a great deal of force. By assuming a half turn position you are preparing your body to transfer this power in one continuous, smooth action.

A second and less obvious purpose of the half turn position occurs when facing your opponent. When viewed from the front, your body seems to be facing forward with shoulders square. However, if someone punches at the center of your chest, the half-turn angle you have

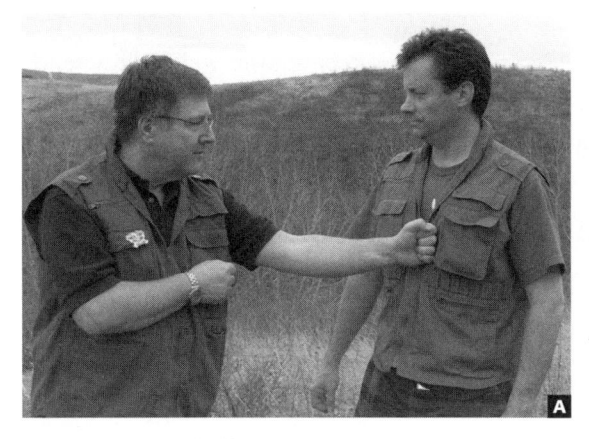

Figure 2-4a. The half turn position causes the punch to slide past the body.

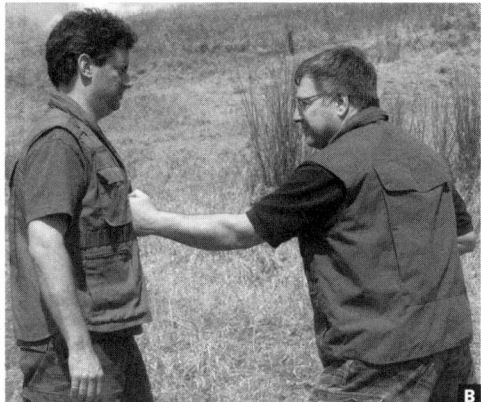

Figure 2-4b. Keeping the upper body square forces you to take the full force of the strike.

assumed will cause the blow to "slip past" on the angle rather than being absorbed by your chest.

When moving from the standing to half turn position, your shoulders should remain level and arm movements small. This prevents your center of gravity from lifting up and upsetting your balance.

## Centering Weight

You will notice in the original illustrations that Jiang Rong Qiao (who posed for the photographs) stands with his weight centered. He does so because centering your weight allows you to move in any direction. For example, you are facing north and your opponent attacks from the southeast. If you are standing with the majority of your weight on the rear leg, you first have to shift your weight forward, centering it, and then turn to face the opponent. This requires two motions.

If your weight is centered, you eliminate the need to shift and can make the turn in only one movement.

While a difference in weight placement may not be that critical on a gym floor and in controlled conditions, it is quite noticeable when done on uneven, cluttered, or slippery ground—the terrain of actual combat.

As we read earlier, Huang states that keeping the weight low tends to reduce power. If your stance is back-weighted, basic biomechanics will show that you will be prevented from delivering all your force into the target.

Having your stance back-weighted also leads to another problem, namely, a tendency to straighten the front leg. Any low kick, such as the xingyi horse kick targeting the straightened knee, would easily cause it to hyperflex, severely damaging it.

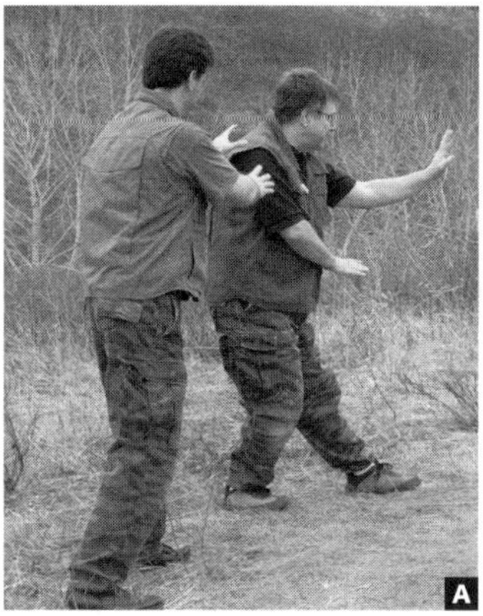

Chapter Two

Figure 2-5a. The opponent attacks while you are in a back-weighted stance.

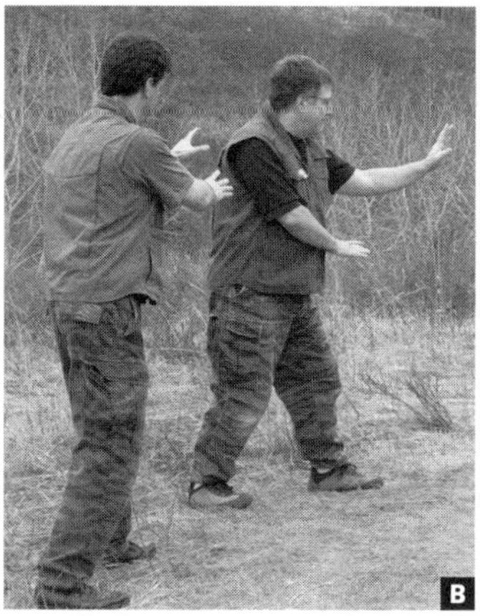

Figure 2-5b. You must shift your weight forward to center it.

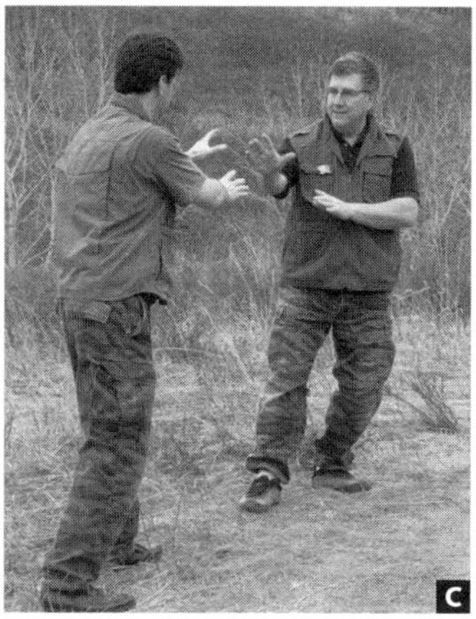

Figure 2-5c. Once your weight is centered, you can turn and defend.

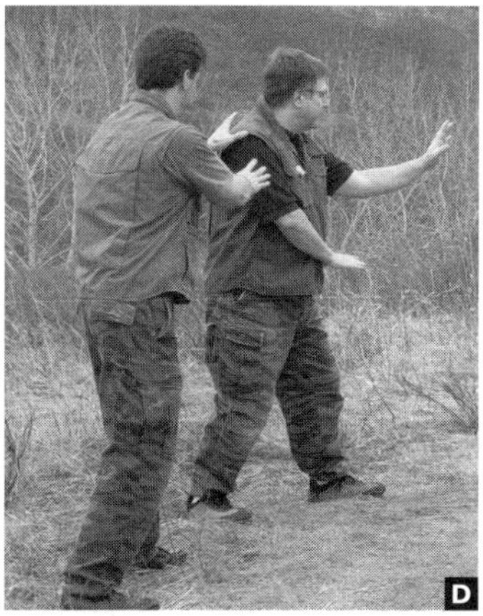

Figure 2-5d. Here your weight is already centered.

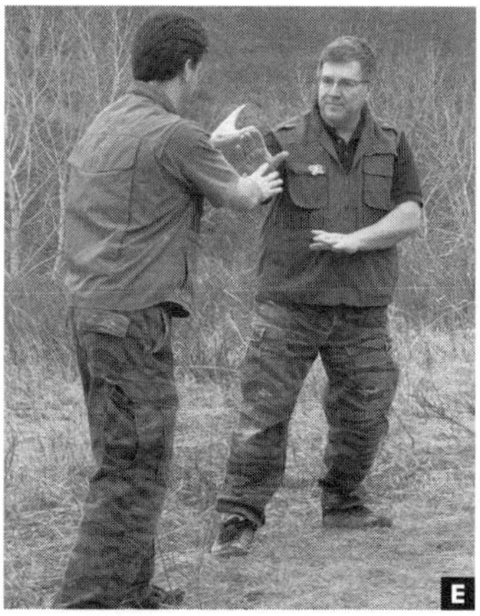

Figure 2-5e. You can immediately turn and defend, eliminating one step in the movement sequence.

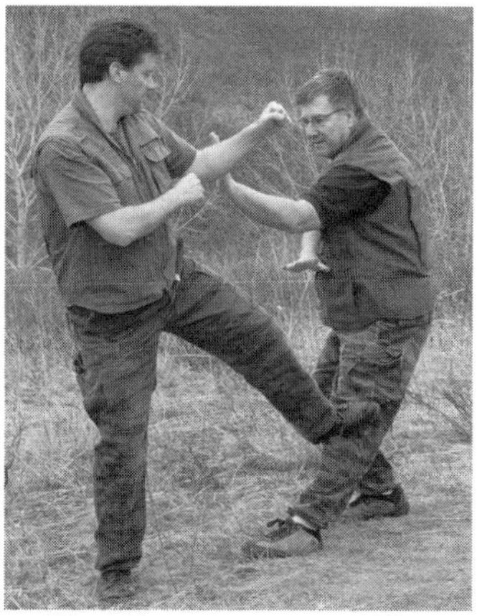

Figure 2-6. A back-weighted stance makes your front knee vulnerable.

## Reinforcing Step

Addition of the reinforcing step at the moment you make contact with the target stabilizes you and helps diminish the likelihood of your force being stopped or redirected back into your body. An analogy to this would be blocking a door after you close it to prevent the wind from pushing it back open.

## Knee and Lead Foot Relationship

In this stance, the knee should face forward while the foot turns in at approximately 5–10 degrees. This relationship increases mechanical efficiency, making the knee more stable and able to better withstand a kick to the knee joint.

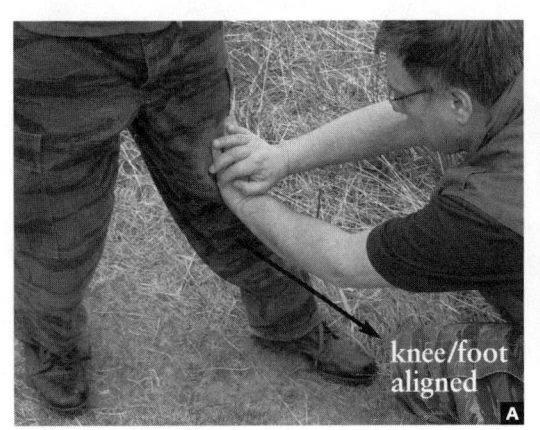

Figure 2-7a. With the foot and knee in alignment, it is easy to cause hyperflexion.

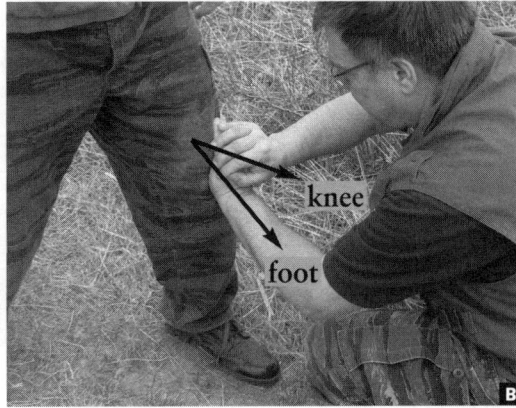

Figure 2-7b. Altering the angle increases mechanical efficiency.

# SECTION IV: SPLITTING FIST ROUTE ILLUSTRATION

The main difference between xingyi and other fist forms lies in the use of the feet. After the front foot moves, the back foot must follow. The fist assists movement of the front foot by coupling with it and causing it to rapidly move forward. Such movement must be reflexive in order to win. Movement of the fist is immediately followed by the back foot vigorously moving up. This creates a springing action from the ground, which pushes the body forward.

> *"If one is capable of doing this, one will be unbeatable."*

This is splitting fist. In *forward stepping method*, three steps form a group:

    Front foot steps forward to become step number one.

    Back foot steps forward to become step number two.

    The foot that steps first follows the second step to become step number three.

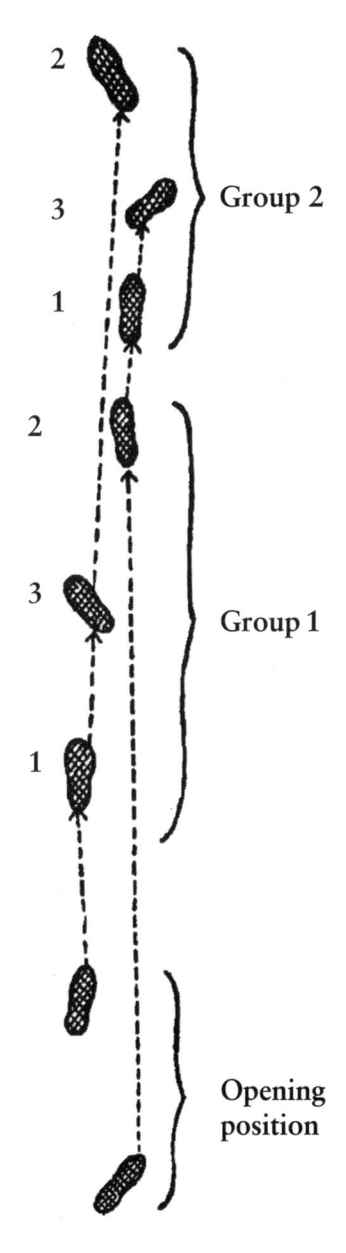

Figure 2-8. Foot pattern.

## SECTION V: ILLUSTRATION OF SPLITTING FIST

To initiate the transition from starting position to splitting fist position, follow the orders:

*"Ready . . . splitting fist . . . forward . . . go."*

**Action #1** (Figure 2-3 again): Change from standing position to opening position.

**Action #2** (Figures 2-9, 2-9m1, and 2-9m2): Change from opening position to starting position.

Clench your fists [hold both your hands tightly], palms facing upward. Both fists rotate out from mouth level. Your little finger faces upward, but not higher than your eyebrows. Back fist follows. Your elbow is in front of your chest. Eyes are level, tongue rolled. Qi sinks.

**Action #3** (Figures 2-10, 2-10m1, and 2-10m2): Change from starting position to *landing position*. Move your front foot first. Back foot follows with a big step forward. Feet and hands land at the same time.

*"In order to be effective, it is important to push fast."*

Back foot follows. Point toe outward. Front foot continues to move forward. The five fingers of the front hand separate and hook. They are level with the heart. The back hand is close to the ribs. Foot, hand, and nose all align.

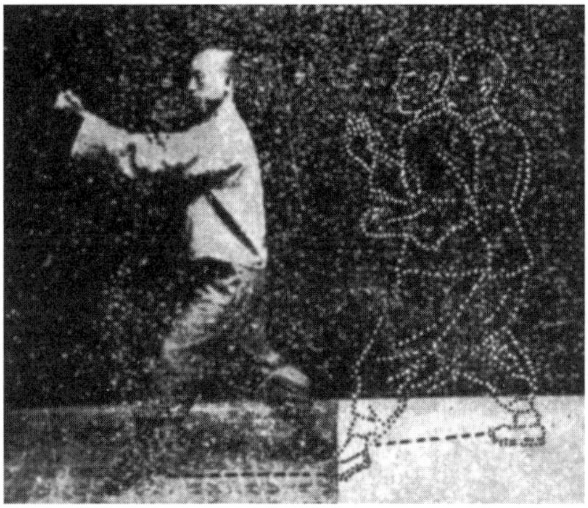

Chapter Two

Figure 2-9.

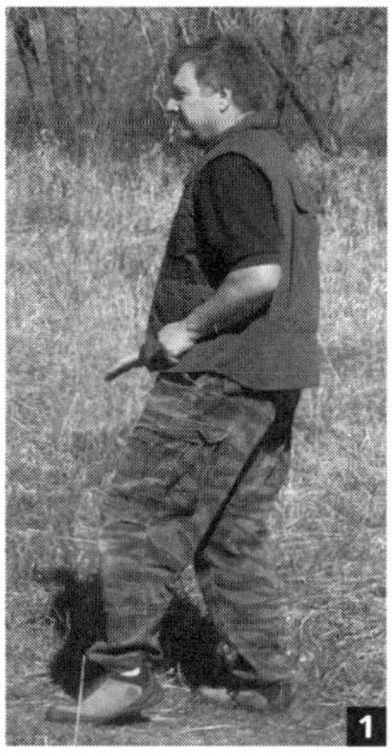

Figure 2-9m1.

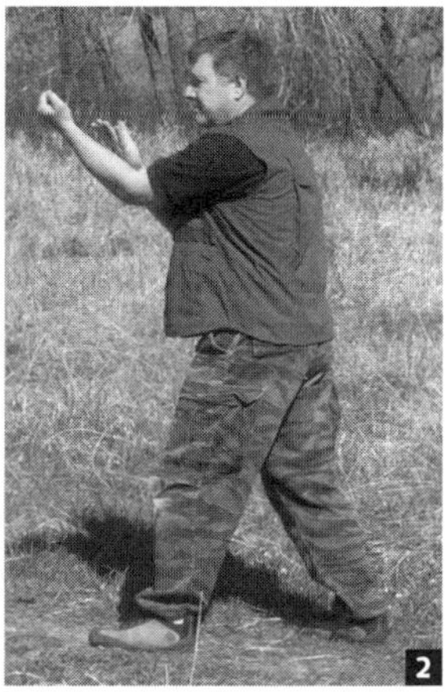

Figure 2-9m2.

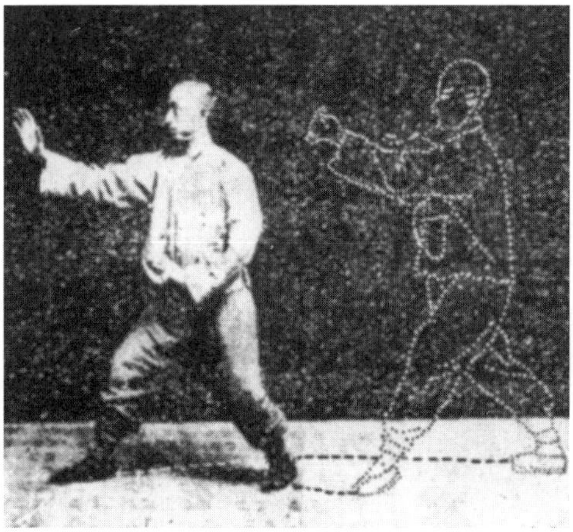

Figure 2-10.

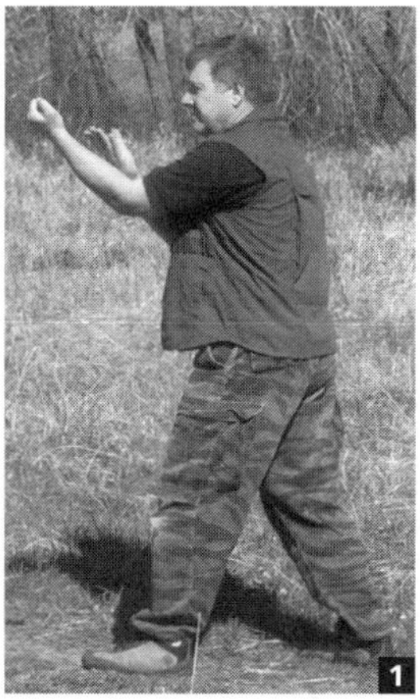

Figure 2-10m1.

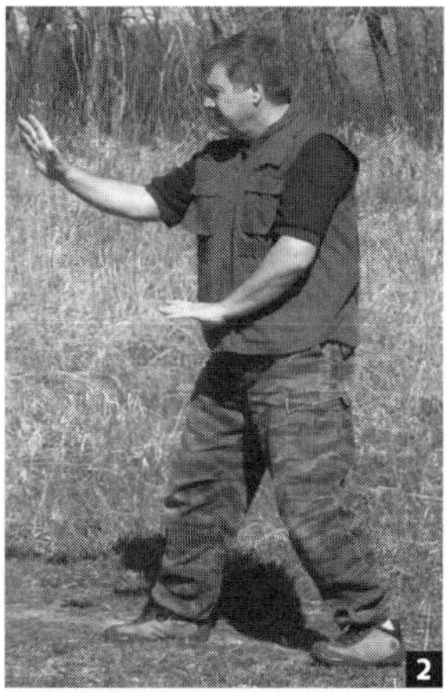

Figure 2-10m2.

## FIRST APPLICATION OF ACTION #2

Simultaneously withdrawing your hand and leg can be used as a counter to a wrist grab. As the opponent seizes your wrist (Figure 2-11a), pull your hand down and back as you shift your weight and withdraw your lead leg (Figure 2-11b). Make sure to keep your upper body and head erect as you lower your center of gravity.

Your downward pulling action will cause the opponent's body to move forward and his head to straighten. His body action indicates he is off balance.

Before he can recover, rotate your wrist, step forward, and punch upward at his face (Figure 2-11c). This will cause his arm to collapse and prevent him from blocking your strike.

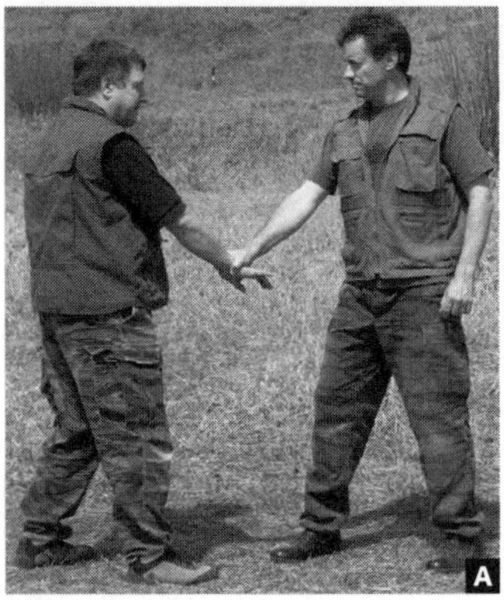

Figure 2-11a.

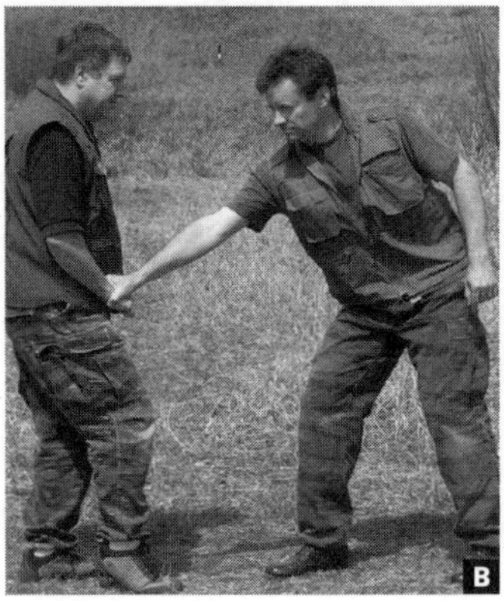

Figure 2-11b.

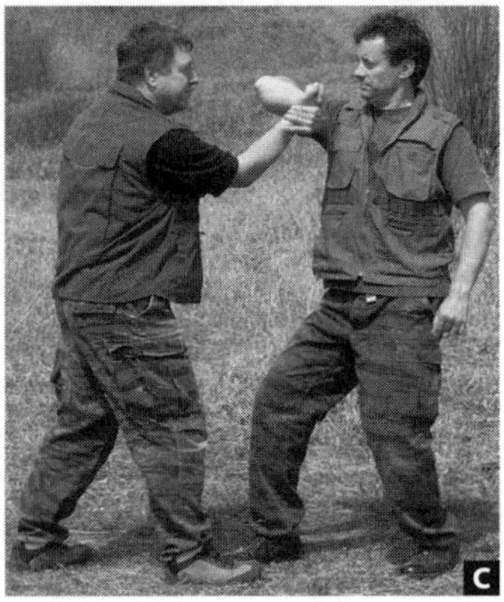

Figure 2-11c.

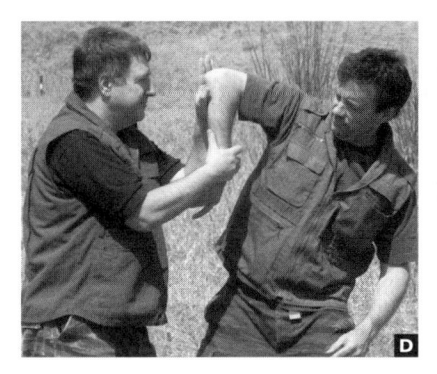

Figure 2-11d. From here you grasp the opponent's elbow and wrist.

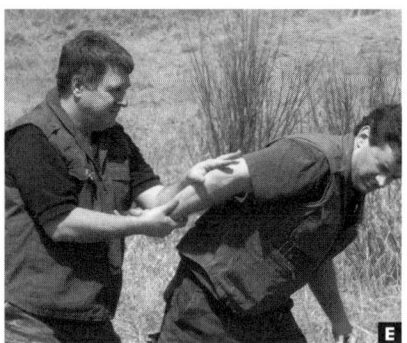

Figure 2-11e. Step forward and apply an arm bar.

## SECOND APPLICATION OF ACTION #2

The uppercut punch in splitting fist is both a block and a punch. It can be used unarmed or with a weapon (such as bayonet or dagger against rifle and bayonet).

Your opponent delivers a straight punch to your chest. You counter by rotating your arm and contacting the outside of his fist and arm (Figure 2-12a). As your arm rotates, deliver an uppercut to his throat or face.

In order to maximize your mechanical efficiency, the angle of your forearm should be greater than 90 degrees with your elbow pointed straight down.

The rotating action of your arm deflects or redirects his punch past your body (Figure 2-12b), setting him up for the counterattack as described in Action #3, below.

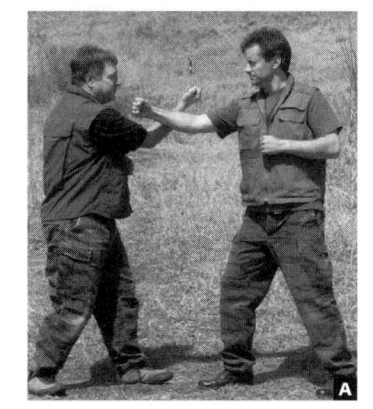

Figure 2-12a.

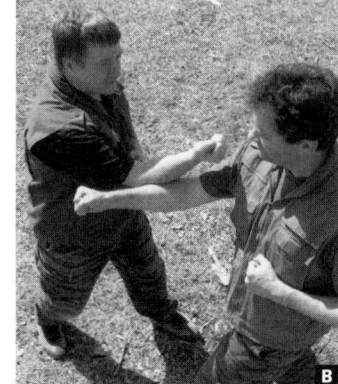

Figure 2-12b.

## ACTION #3: COUNTERATTACK USING THE LANDING POSITION

The landing position consists of two parts: the overturning and downward movement of your lead hand, and the step through and strike.

In splitting fist there are two methods of delivering the follow-up strike. The first and older method (pre-1920s) uses a *yin palm* with fingers extended. The second, more "contemporary" method (after the mid-1920s) is the one illustrated in Huang's book. Here the palm is vertical and the strike is delivered with a quick rotational snapping action of the wrist at the moment of impact.

While both strikes follow the overturning and downward movement of the lead arm, their applications are different. Of the two, Huang's method is potentially more lethal and was the one advocated by Sun Lu Tang and taught to the Chinese army.

Figure 2-13a.

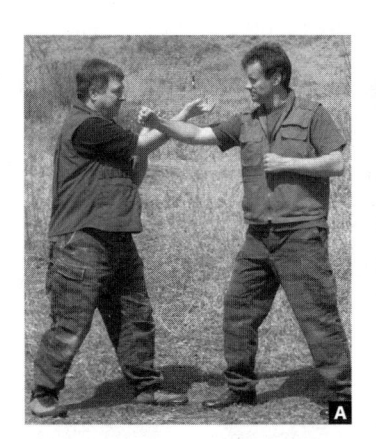

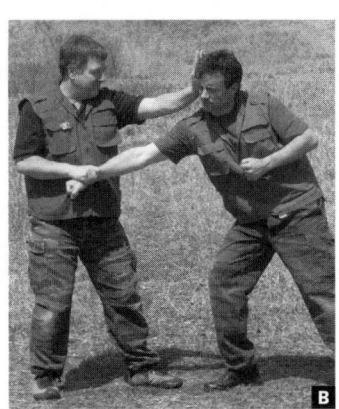

Figure 2-13b.

## APPLICATION OF THE NECK BREAK

Once you have blocked your attacker's punch, grasp his arm and use the overturning action of your arm to pull him forward and down (Figure 2-13a).

As he comes forward, strike him with your vertical palm (Figure 2-13b). These two simultaneous actions create a whiplash effect, driving his head backward. The force, if applied properly, can break his neck.

# SECTION VI: TURNING AROUND IN SPLITTING FIST

To turn around while in forward stepping position, follow the orders:

"Stop . . . . to the back . . . turn."

As soon as the order "stop" is given, stop all action. When you hear "to the back," note which hand is in front. If your left hand is in front, turn to the right. If right hand is in front, turn left. This turn causes your front foot to become the back foot, and vice versa.

Using the *group theory (grouping of steps)* we see:

Front foot steps forward to become step number one.

Back foot steps forward to become step number two.

The foot that stepped first now follows to become step number three.

*(The foot pattern for turning is shown in Figure 2-14.)*

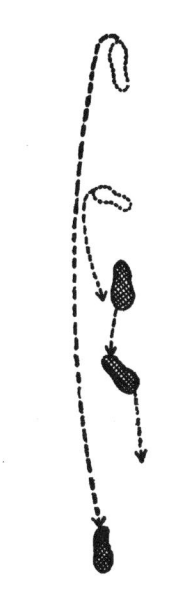

Figure 2-14. Foot pattern for turning.

# SECTION VII: DRILLING FIST ROUTE ILLUSTRATION

*Drilling fist's forward route (forward stepping pattern)* is the same as that of splitting fist. As with splitting fist, three steps form one group.

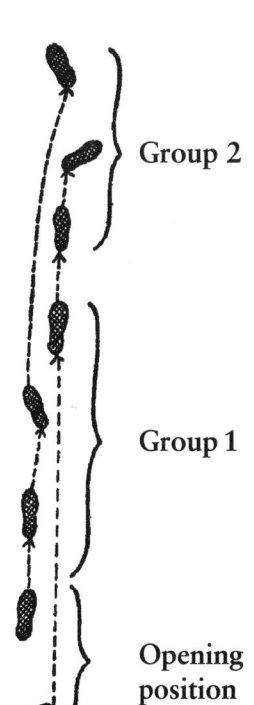

Figure 2-15. Foot pattern.

## SECTION VIII: ILLUSTRATION OF DRILLING FIST

To change from standing position to drilling fist position, follow the orders:

*"Ready . . . drilling fist . . . forward . . . go."*

**Action #1:** When you hear this order, change to opening position (Figure 2-3).

**Action #2** (Figures 2-16 and 2-16m): Change from opening position to starting position. As you step forward with your left foot, turn the left hand upward. Your palm and elbow should be slightly bent, like a bow. Right hand forms a fist, and faces upward, lightly touching your ribs. Look beyond your lead hand.

**Action #3** (Figures 2-17 and 2-17m): Move from Action #2 to landing position. After the left foot opening is complete, step forward with your right foot. Strike out with your fist as the foot lands. Simultaneously, retract your left fist and position it near your right elbow. Left foot follows with toes out. Right foot is straight. Front fist should appear as if you are punching the enemy's nose. Legs, feet, hands, and nose must align properly. All stepping is done according to the orders. From this position change to Action #2 and continue the stepping sequences by alternating.

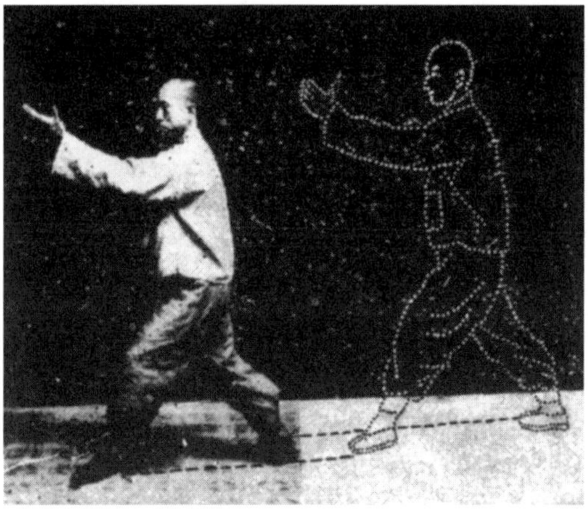

Chapter Two    **29**

Figure 2-16.

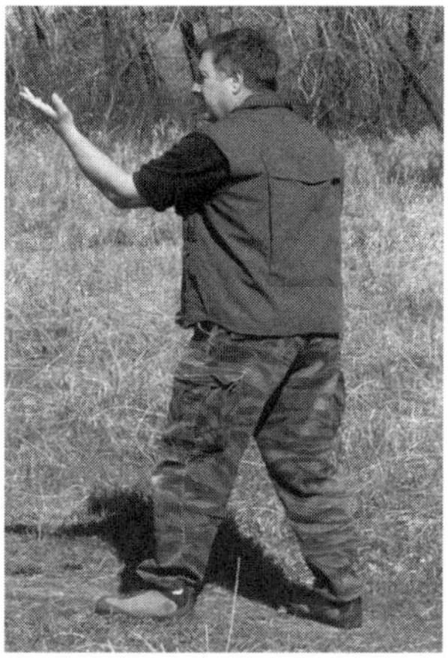

Figure 2-16m.

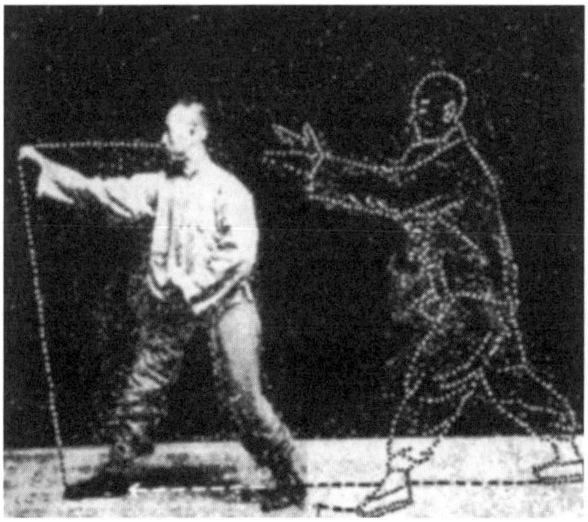

Figure 2-17.

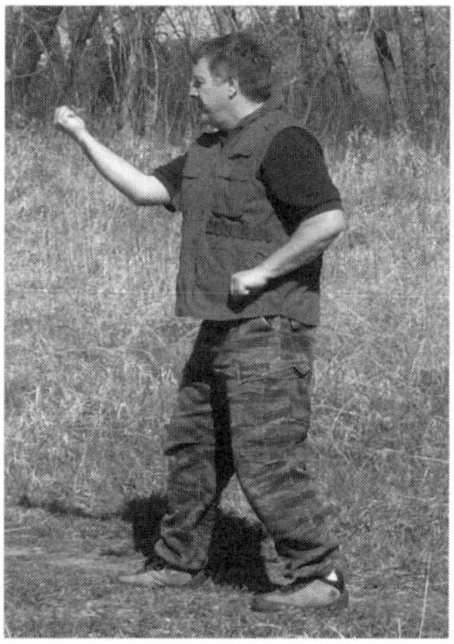

Figure 2-17m.

## APPLICATIONS OF DRILLING FIST
### First Application of Action #3

As we saw in splitting, the uppercut can be used as either a block or a punch. Here, however, the counterattack is somewhat different.

Your opponent attacks with a punch. As he punches, use your drilling fist to block (Figure 2-18a). Step in and deliver a second drilling fist to his exposed side (Figures 2-18b and 2-18c).

Target areas include the intercostal nerves between the ribs, the armpit, and the muscle under the back of the shoulder joint.

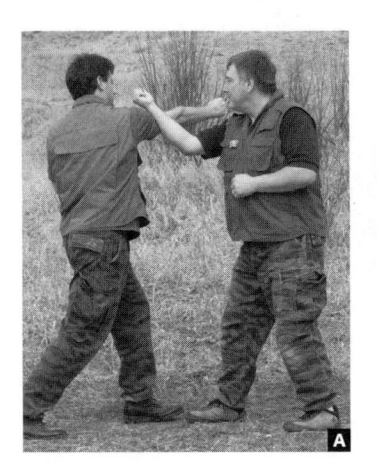

Figure 2-18a.

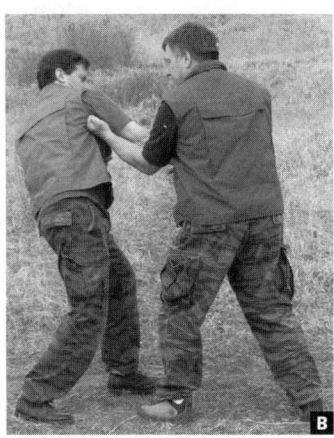

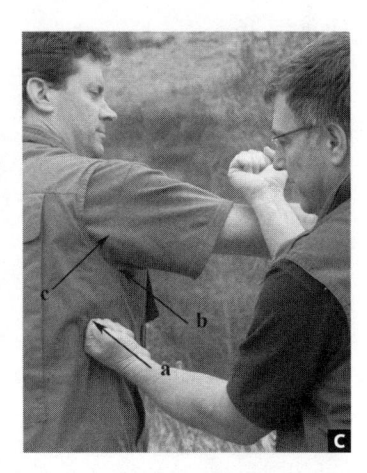

Figure 2-18b.

Figure 2-18c: Target areas include (a) intercostal nerves, (b) armpit, and (c) the muscle under the shoulder joint.

## Second Application of Action #3

In the first two-person fixed training form taught at the Central Military Academy, the retracting hand is often used to hook the opponent's lead arm in order to pull him off balance. For example, your opponent attacks with a straight punch aimed at your midsection.

Hook the punch as you retract your hand and pull his arm slightly past you (Figure 2-19a). Immediately counter with a punch (Figure 2-19b) to the base of his sternum, the area under the right nipple, or the throat (Figure 2-19c). Striking any of these areas with full force can cause severe damage or even death.

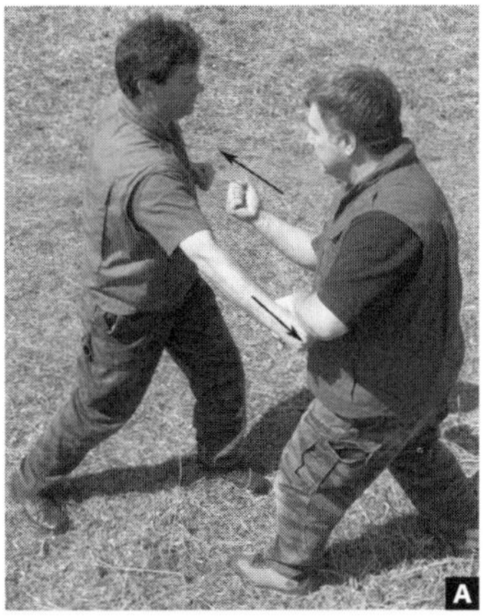

Figure 2-19a.

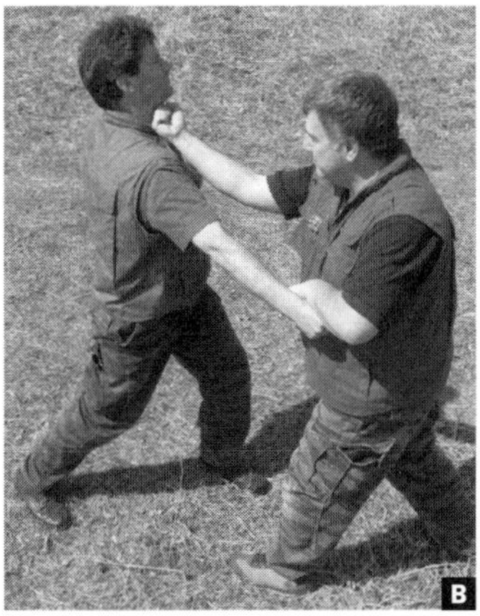

Figure 2-19b.

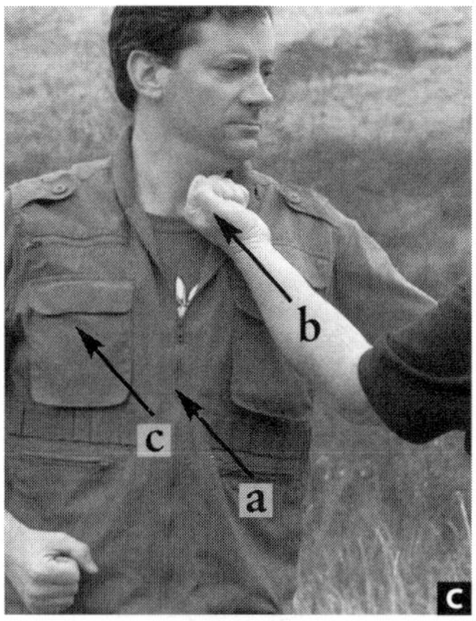

Figure 2-19c: Target areas include (a) base of sternum, (b) area under right nipple, and (c) the throat.

## Third Application of Action #3

In this example, your attacker uses a dagger or bayonet to stab your midsection (Figure 2-20a).

As he thrusts, use your retracting hand to hook his weapon hand (Figure 2-20b) and pull it forward and past your body (Figure 2-20c). Counter by punching or grabbing his throat (Figure 2-20d). If the opponent closes distance as he thrusts, you may have to perform a withdrawing step (Figure 2-20e), as in splitting fist, in order to allow the weapon to clear your body.

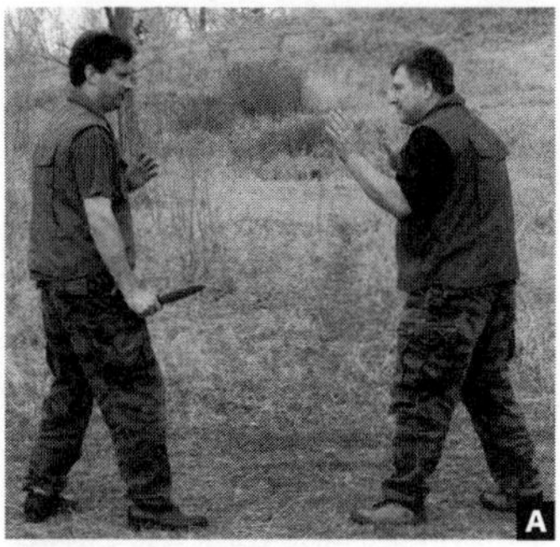

Figure 2-20a.

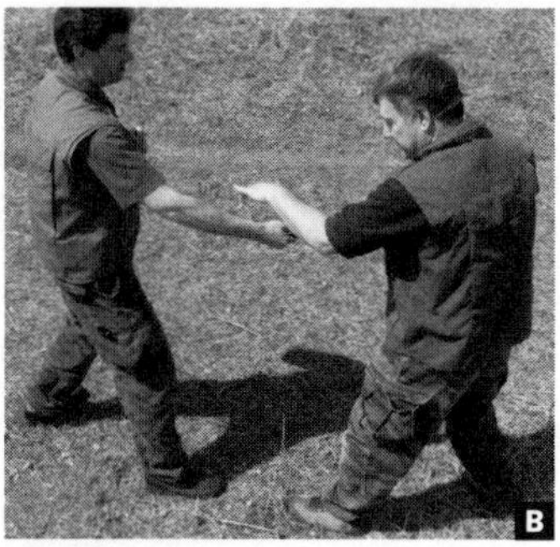

Figure 2-20b.

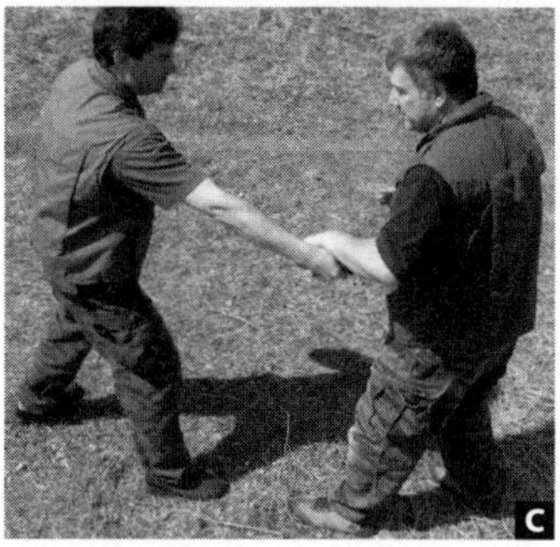

Figure 2-20c.

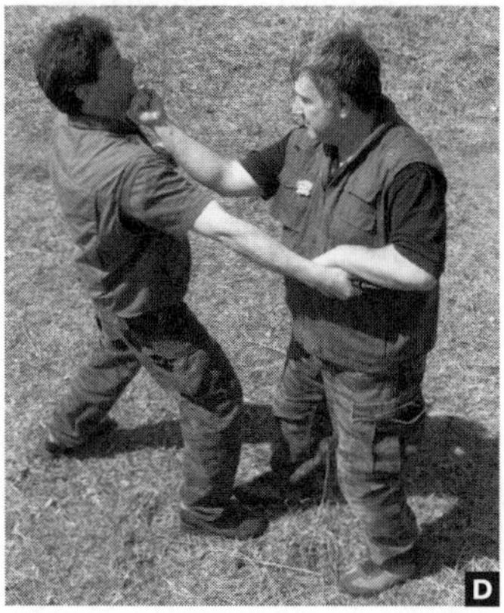

Figure 2-20d.

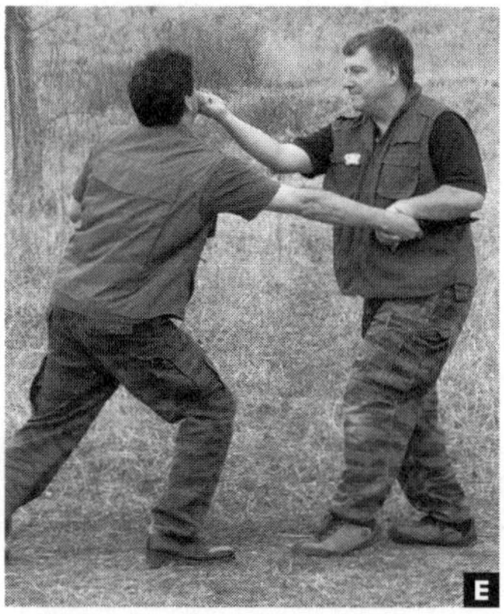

Figure 2-20e.

# SECTION IX: TURNING AROUND IN DRILLING FIST

To turn around from forward stepping position, follow the orders:

*"Stop . . . to the back . . . turn."*

When you hear "stop," cease all action. When you hear "to the back . . . turn," note whether your right or left hand is in front. If your right hand is in front, turn from the left to the back. If your left hand is in front, make a right turn to the back. Your right hand moves next to your ribs and turns over in order to catch the enemy's wrist. Stepping is the same as in splitting fist.

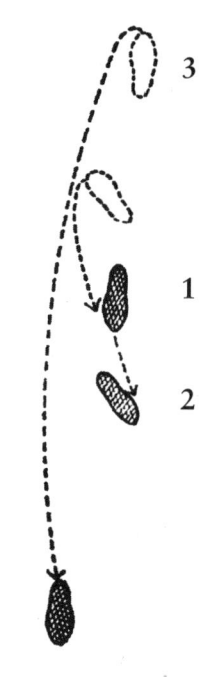

Figure 2-21. Foot pattern of drilling fist and turning.

# SECTION X: CRUSHING FIST ROUTE ILLUSTRATION

Crushing fist is considered simple because there is no difference between starting and landing pose. Turning around, however, is more complicated than in other fist forms. This is why *forward position* and *body turning position* are practiced separately.

Because this movement is complex, practice the body turning position in sections. The standard method of practice is to have your left foot in front and right foot following from behind. This method is known as *left foot crushing fist*.

Opening position

Figure 2-22. Foot pattern of crushing fist.

## SECTION XI: TURNING AROUND IN CRUSHING FIST

To change from the standing position to the crushing fist position, follow the order:

*"Ready . . . crushing fist."*

**Action #1:** Upon hearing the order, change to opening position (Figure 2-3).

**Action #2** (Figures 2-23, 2-23m1, and 2-23m2): Immediately change to forward stepping position. First move your left foot forward. Follow with your right foot. Keep your right ankle and left heel side by side, but not close together. Bend legs to about 120 degrees. Keep upper body straight. Tightly clench both hands and rotate your rear hand forward and back.

Figure 2-23.

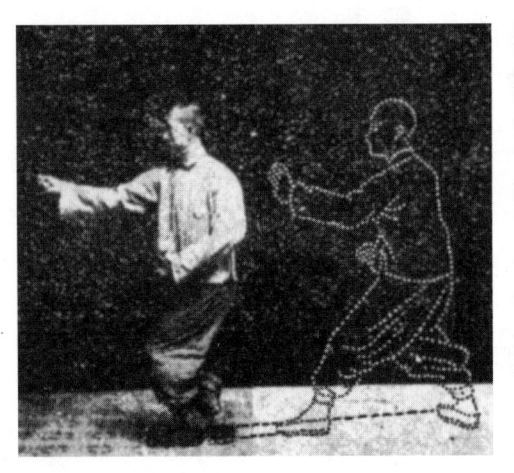

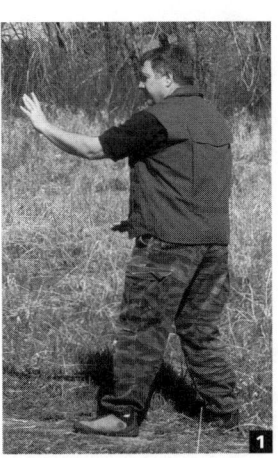

Figure 2-23m1.

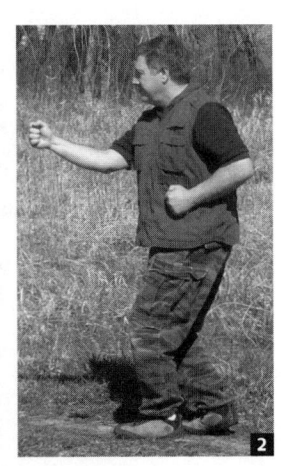

Figure 2-23m2.

## INCREASING MECHANICAL EFFICIENCY

The crushing fist method uses a vertical fist, which is the most mechanically efficient way to punch. Why is this punch so efficient?

First, the elbows are pointed downward and close to the body with the angle of the arm slightly upward (approximately 15 degrees from the horizontal). This elbow position and angle increases your leverage.

Second, in crushing fist, the punch travels along your side to a point that is in alignment with the center line of your body. This alignment combines the force of your arm with the weight of your body. As you step forward, your body weight becomes part of the punch and significantly increases the total amount of force behind the blow.

In contrast, a punch delivered straight out from your shoulder relies solely on arm strength for its power. Little or no body weight is included, making this type of punch less efficient.

A simple way to test this is to stand with your fist out in the crushing fist position just described. Have someone place both hands on your fist and lean with full weight against you. Try to both support the person and push him backward.

Next, use a horizontal punch with your shoulders square and repeat the procedure. You will find that it is easier to support the weight with elbows down and aligned with your body.

## Consistent Strikes

The ability to consistently and accurately strike a target is a necessary skill in close combat. Pounding fist is designed to develop this skill.

When performing the vertical punches, the hand that is outstretched is lowered slightly prior to retraction. The next punch comes over the top of this punch and the bottom of this fist rubs against the top of the one you just lowered. Alternating punches in this manner ensures that the beginner will develop an ability to consistently strike the same point in space.

## Application

Your opponent throws a roundhouse kick (Figure 2-24a). Immediately step in and punch (Figure 2-24b).

Because the force of his kick is concentrated at his foot, the closer you move toward his knee, the less force your body has to absorb, thus making his kick ineffective.

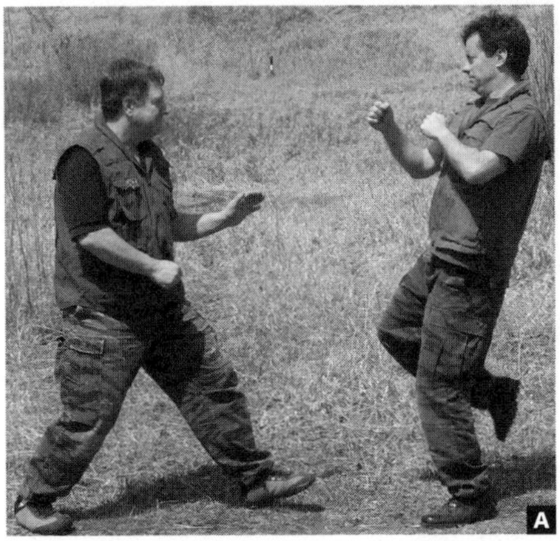

Figure 2-24a.

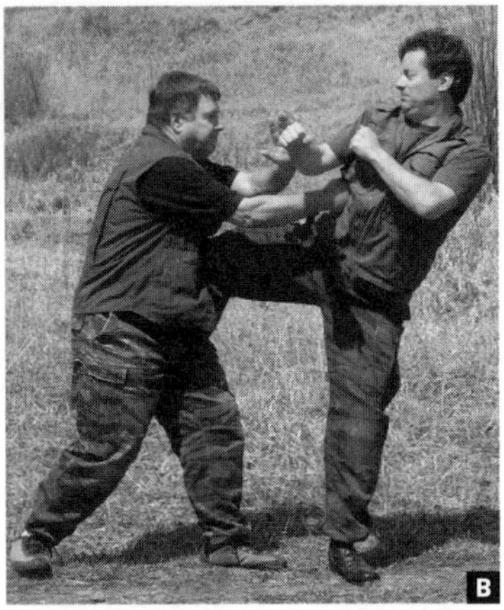

Figure 2-24b.

# ACTION #3: MOVING FROM ACTION #2 INTO THE TURNING POSITION

Use your left foot to cross step to the right. Utilize the momentum of this movement, and turn to the back. Lift your right foot. Stretch out right hand with palm upward. Turn your left fist upward and push out with force. As your feet and hands land simultaneously, stretch both palms straight out and change to yin palm. Stretch your elbows and align palms with chest. The wrist of your back hand lightly touches your right side [ribs].

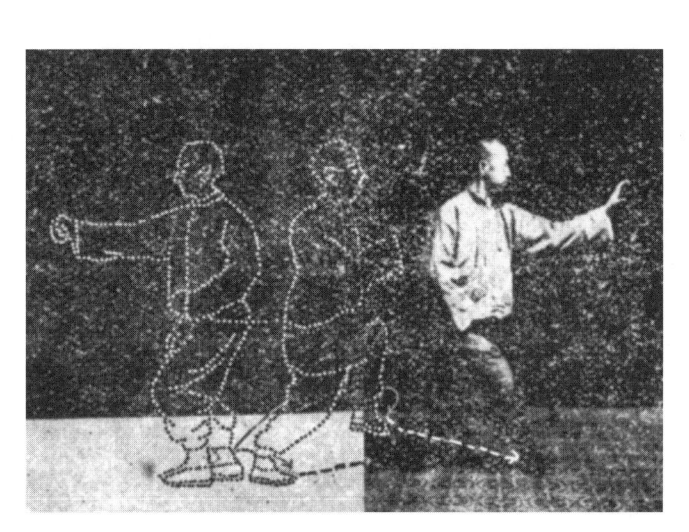

Figure 2-25.

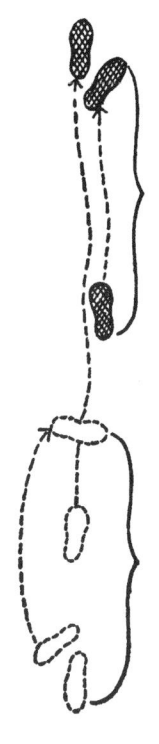

Figure 2-26. Foot pattern of Action #3.

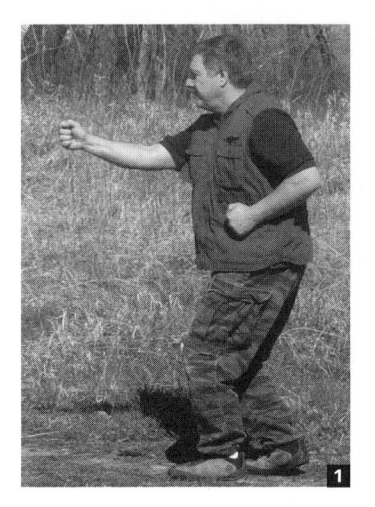

Figure 2-25m1.

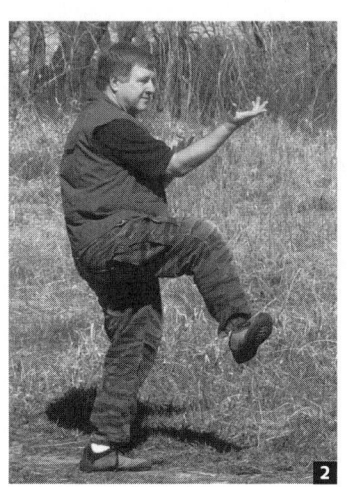

Figure 2-25m2.

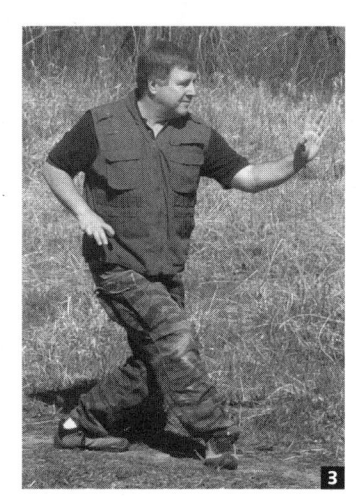

Figure 2-25m3.

## APPLICATIONS OF ACTION #3

The turning action described by Huang is similar in appearance and application to *dragon* in the twelve animal forms. For example, your opponent attacks with a straight punch or a punch-kick combination.

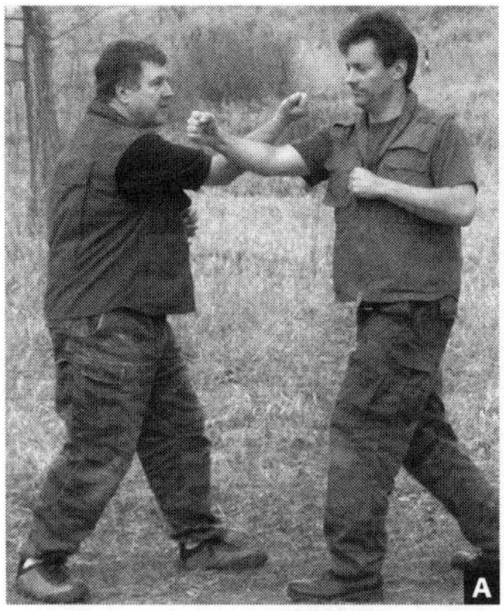

Figure 2-27a. If the opponent punches use your lead hand to block.

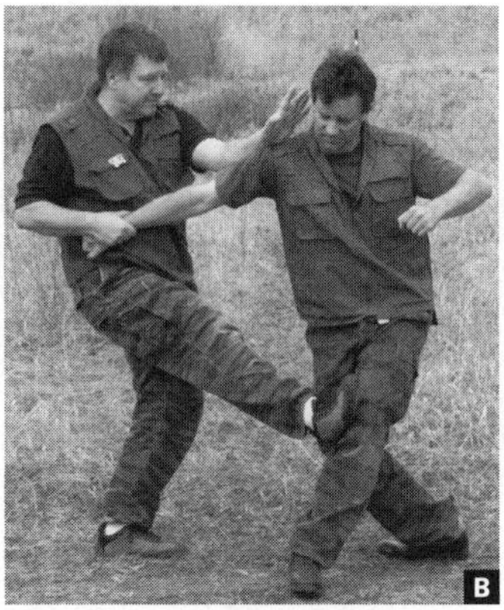

Figure 2-27b. Immediately kick his leg or knee.

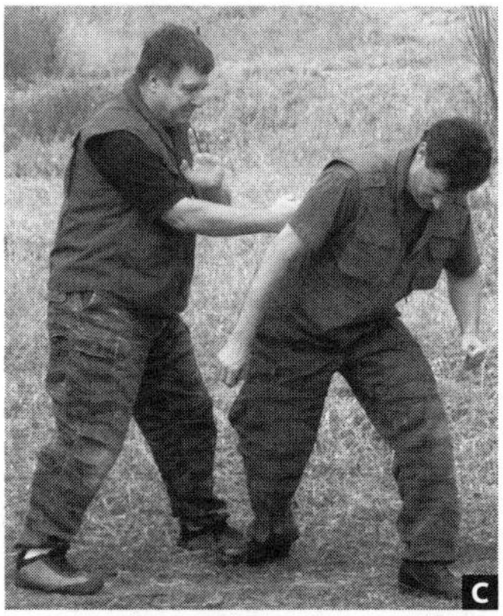

Figure 2-27c. Follow up with another punch.

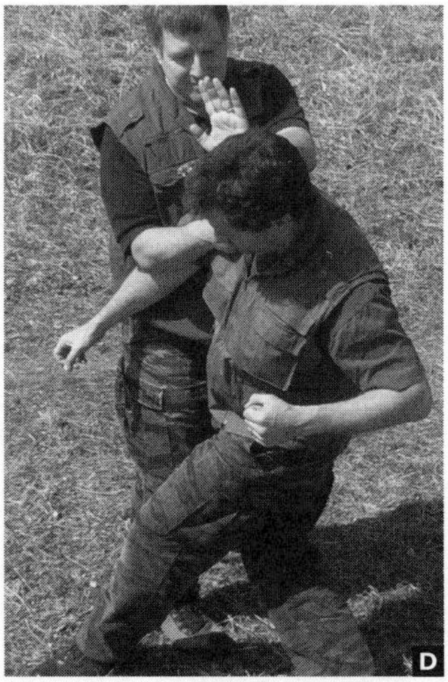

Figure 2-27d. Alternately, strike the side of his neck and face.

If the opponent kicks first, use your heel to strike his shin (Figure 2-28).

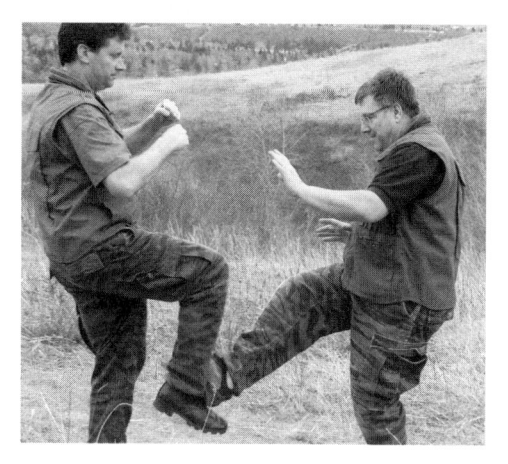

Figure 2-28.

Another option is to reach around the opponent's head and use your punching action to trap his head (Figures 2-29a to 2-29c).

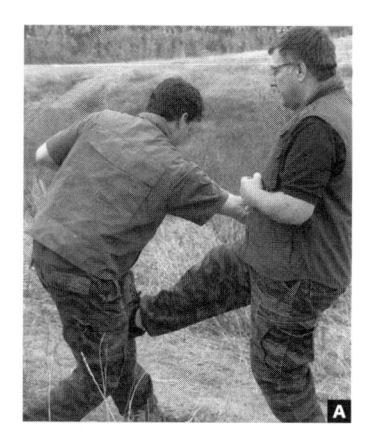

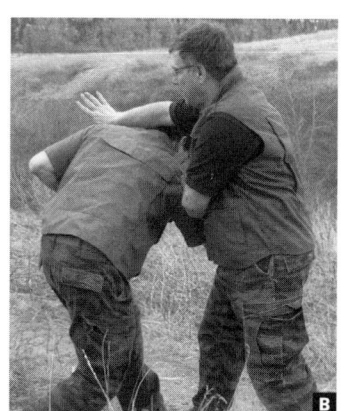

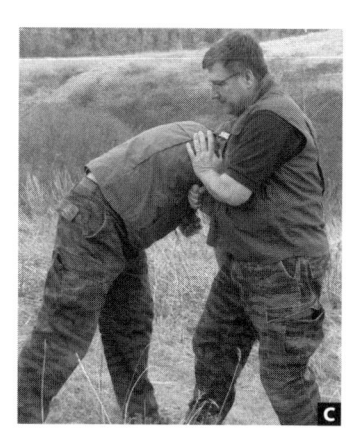

Figure 2-29a.  Figure 2-29b.  Figure 2-29c.

## SECTION XII: POUNDING FIST ROUTE ILLUSTRATION

In splitting fist, three steps form a group.

In crushing fist, two steps form a group.

In pounding fist, four steps form a group.

The style of forward movement for pounding fist is diagonal (Figure 2-30).

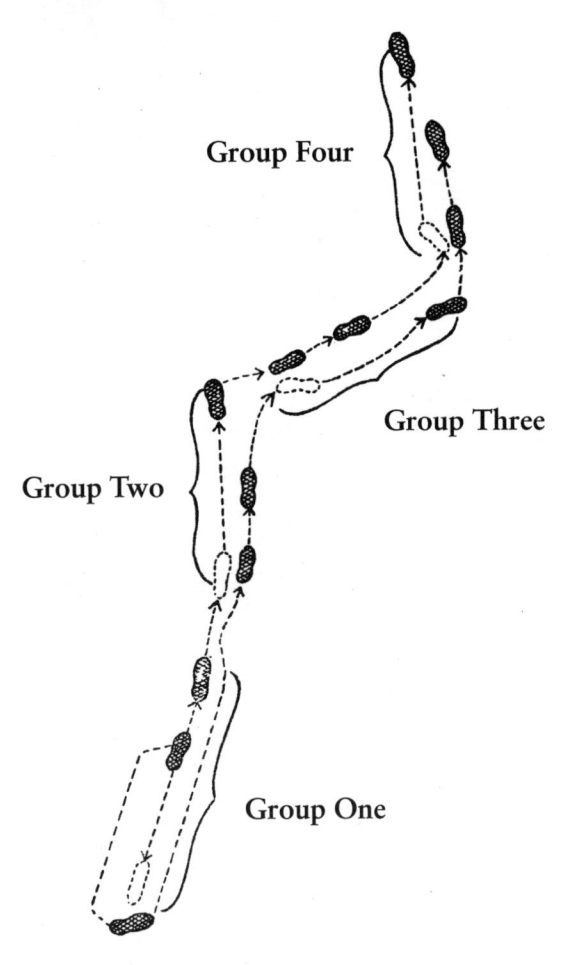

Figure 2-30. Foot pattern of pounding fist.

# SECTION XIII: ILLUSTRATION OF POUNDING FIST

To change from standing position to pounding fist position, follow the orders:

*"Ready . . . pounding fist."*

**Action #1:** When the order is heard, change to opening position (Figure 2-3).

**Action #2** (Figures 2-31, 2-31m1, and 2-31m2): Quickly change to starting position.

First, step forward with your left foot. Follow with the right foot, stepping diagonally. Your eyes and face look slightly to the left. Both your hands form fists. Palms face upward, touching the abdomen in a "T." Hold your elbows tightly to the sides of your body.

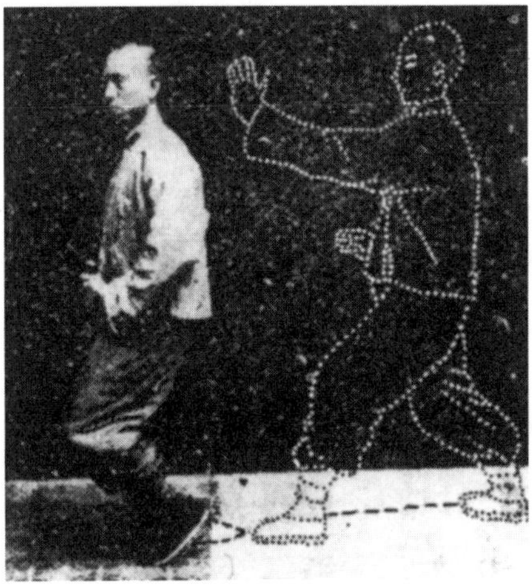

Figure 3-31.

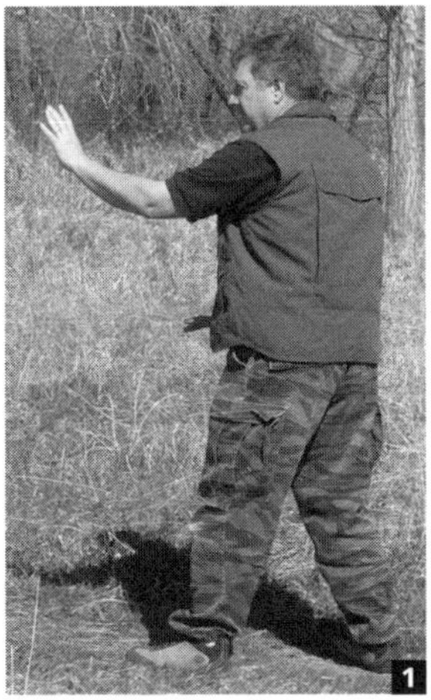

Figure 3-31m1.

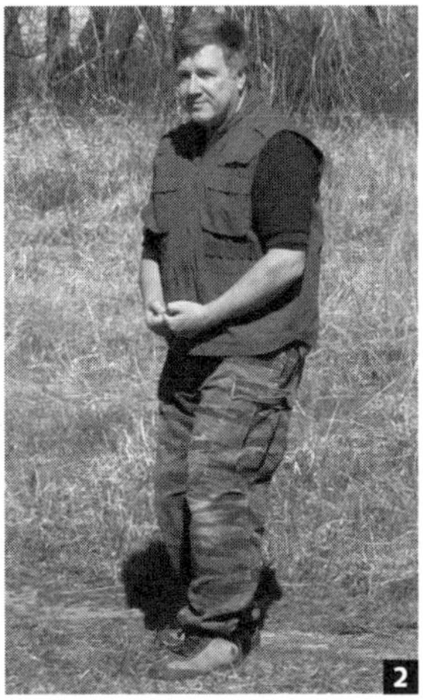

Figure 3-31m2.

**Action #3** (Figures 2-32 and 2-32m): Immediately change to landing position. Use your right hand to punch out with force. Eyes are level. Left foot is forward. As you punch, turn your left fist upward and place it above your eyebrow. Alternate left and right sides as you move forward.

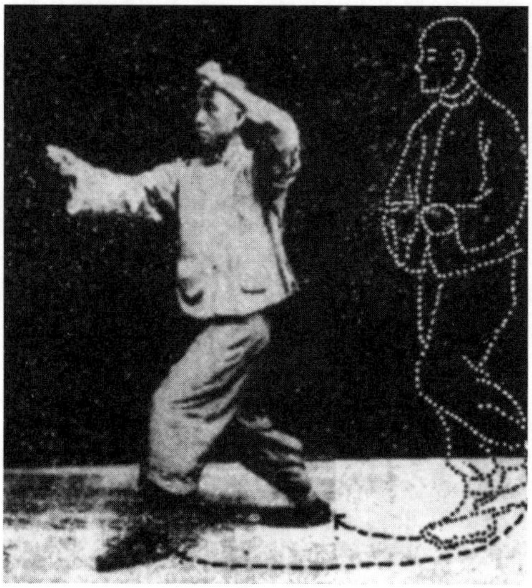

Figure 2-32.

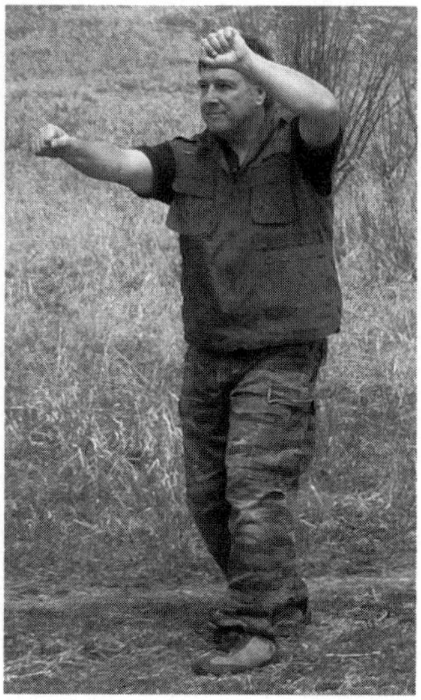

Figure 2-32m.

## APPLICATION AGAINST AN EMPTY HAND ATTACK

When teaching empty hand combat, the Chinese army had a saying:

*"Every strike is a block and every block a strike."*

Pounding fist is no exception.

As your opponent attempts to strike your upper body or torso, use the stepping action and rotational movement of your arm to block and redirect his attack past your body (Figure 2-33a). If done properly, your action will throw him completely off balance, allowing you to deliver a counterpunch in one continuous motion.

If done from the outside, lift his arm to expose his armpit or side of the body (Figure 2-33b).

If done from the inside, strike his shoulder, face, or throat.

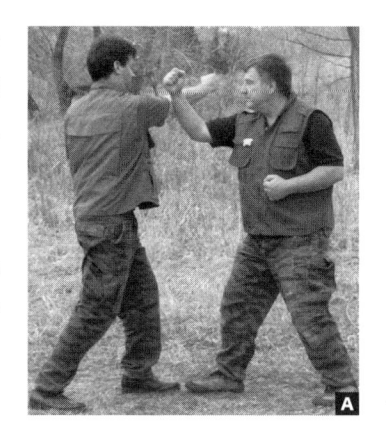

Figure 2-33a.

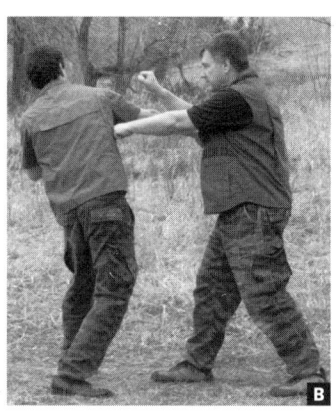

Figure 2-33b.

## APPLICATION AGAINST A KNIFE ATTACK

Your opponent holds the knife in the reverse grip (Figure 2-34a). As he cuts to your face, use your lead arm to come under the attack and grab his wrist (Figure 2-34b). Quickly rotate your hand. This will cause the knife to pop out of his grip. As you pull, deliver your punch (Figure 2-34c).

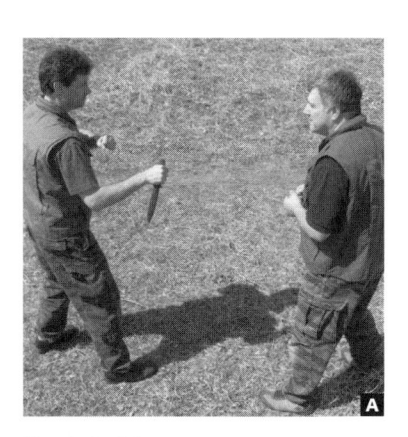

Figure 2-34a.

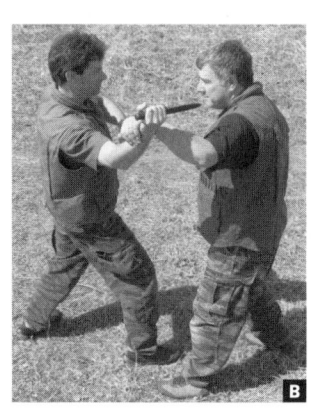

Figure 2-34b.

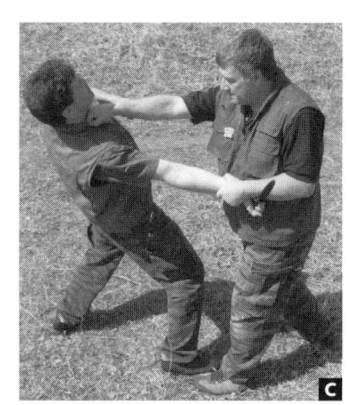

Figure 2-34c.

## SECTION XIV: TURNING AROUND IN POUNDING FIST

To turn around while in forward stepping position, follow the orders:

*"Stop . . . to the back . . . turn."*

When you hear the command, turn from the left if left hand is in front. If your right hand is in front, turn from the right toward the back.

As you turn, your left foot moves slightly and your right foot takes the left foot's position. Next, lift the right foot and move it 180 degrees [north/south]. If your front diagonal position is in the southeast direction, you will turn around and strike in the northeast direction. (Although this theory can be applied to all four corners, only one example is shown in Figure 2-35.)

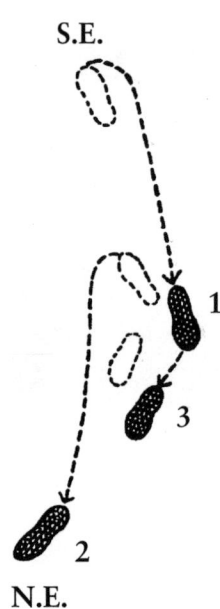

Figure 2-35. Foot pattern of pounding fist and turning.

## SECTION XV: CROSSING FIST ROUTE ILLUSTRATION

Crossing fist also utilizes diagonal stepping. Its foot pattern resembles both splitting fist and drilling fist. However, crossing fist is not done in a straight line. Its diagonal [curved] pattern is also similar to that of pounding fist, but there are fewer steps.

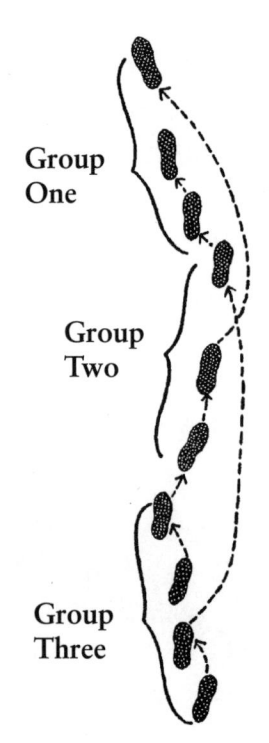

Figure 2-36. Foot pattern of crossing fist.

# SECTION XVI: ILLUSTRATION OF CROSSING FIST

To change from standing position to crossing fist position, follow the orders:

*"Ready . . . crossing fist . . . forward . . . go."*

**Action #1:** Move into opening position by making a half turn to the right (Figure 2-3).

**Action #2** (Figures 2-37, 2-37m1, and 2-37m2): Continuing from Action #1, change to the starting position.

Figure 2-37.

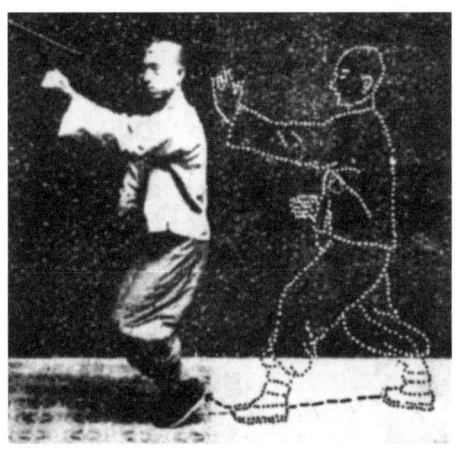

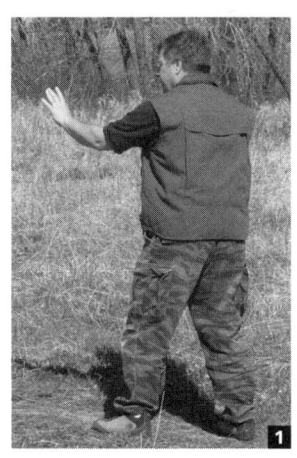

Figure 2-37m1.

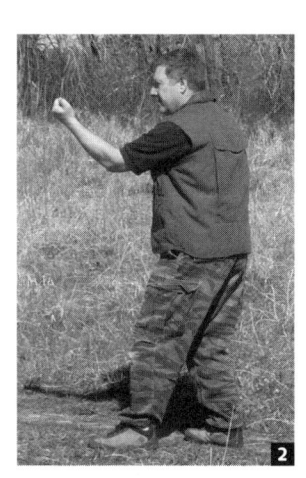

Figure 2-37m2.

Lift your front foot and move it so that it is together with the back foot. As this occurs, straighten the back leg and make both hands into fists. Your front fist faces upward, at eye level. Back fist is held tight to the body, below the line of the elbow. Body is straight. Eyes are level.

**Action #3** (Figures 2-38 and 2-38m): In order to change from starting position to landing position, step forward with your left foot and turn to the left, using a half face body position. At the same time turn your right fist so your little finger faces upwards. Use your *(right)* fist to strike straight out, level with the eyes. Keep elbows slightly bent. Withdraw your left fist and keep it level with the elbow. Alternate the action left to right as you move forward. Crossing fist is called the *horizontal fist* because the lower fist strikes out in a horizontal direction.

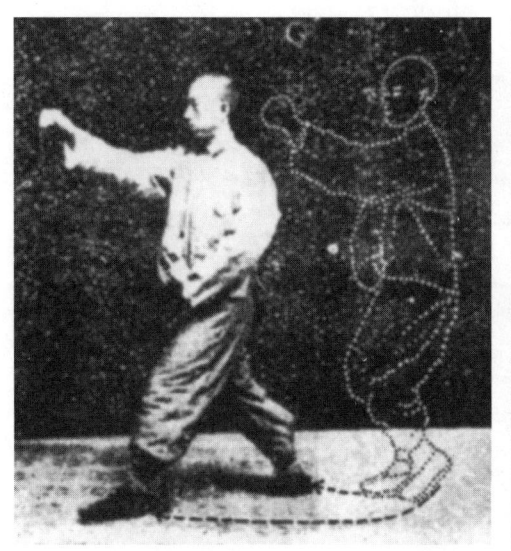

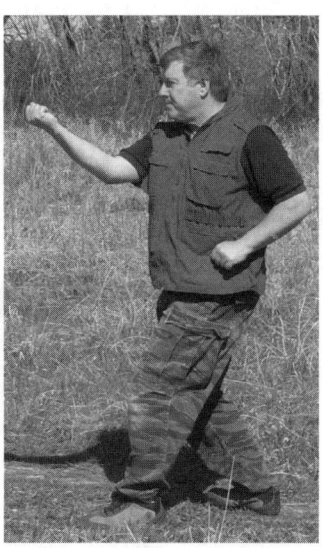

Figure 2-38.

Figure 2-38m.

## SECTION XVII: TURNING AROUND IN CROSSING FIST

To turn around from the forward stepping position, follow the orders:

*"Stop . . . to the back . . . turn."*

When you hear "stop," stop all action. When you hear the order to turn, note which foot is forward. If your left foot is in front, turn to the right. If right foot is in front, use your left foot to turn to the back. As you turn to the left, slightly move the left foot. Move your right foot forward and once again move your left foot forward. Your fist drills and right foot follows.

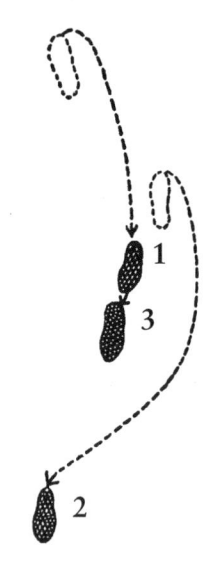

Figure 2-39. Foot pattern for crossing fist and turning.

## SECTION XVIII: EXPLANATION OF LINKING FIST'S OPENING AND STEPPING DIAGRAM

The opening movement of linking fist is the same as that of five element fist. In addition to right half turn position and opening pose, linking fist is further divided into ten actions or movements. (The foot pattern is illustrated in Figure 2-40.)

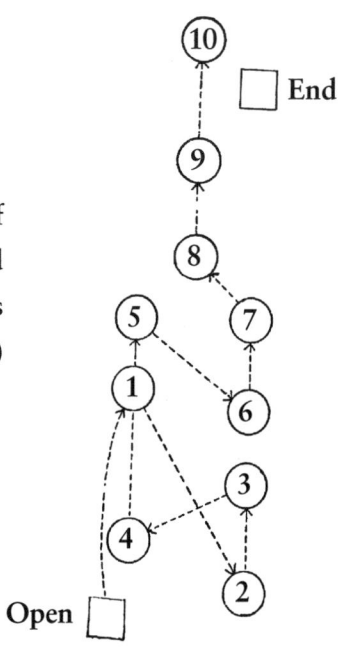

Figure 2-40. Foot pattern of linking fist.

## SECTION XIX: ILLUSTRATION OF LINKING FIST

To make the transition from standing position to linking fist, follow the orders:

*"Ready . . . link . . . forward . . . go."*

**Action #1** (Figures 2-41, 2-41m1, and 2-41m2): When the word "link" is heard, change to opening position. When "go" is heard, make both hands into fists. Step forward with your left foot. Punch straight out from the chest with your right fist. As your right hand strikes out, draw your left fist back near the stomach. Palms should face upward. Right foot follows and steps forward, so your ankle aligns with the heel of your left foot. Slightly bend both legs and tilt your hips.

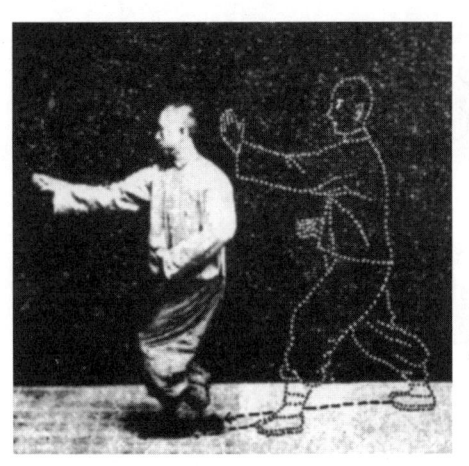

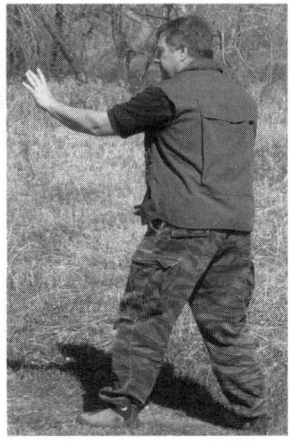

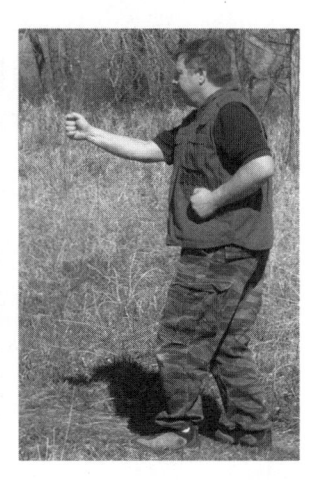

Figure 2-41.

Figure 2-41m1.

Figure 2-41m2.

**Action #2** (Figures 2-42 and 2-42m): Step diagonally to the right with your right leg. Foot lands horizontally. Immediately follow this with a large (diagonal) backward step with your left foot. Feet land approximately 12 inches apart. Step back with right foot. *(This transition move is not shown in the original photograph.)* Both hands still retain their original position. As your left foot lands, withdraw the right fist and place it near the stomach. Immediately punch out with your left fist. This aligns it with your chest to form a scissor-like position known as *scissor-stepping*.

**Action #3** (Figures 2-43 and 2-43m): Step forward with right leg. Right fist follows by punching outward and lining up with your chest. Draw left fist back near the stomach. Turn palms upward. Move left foot slightly forward.

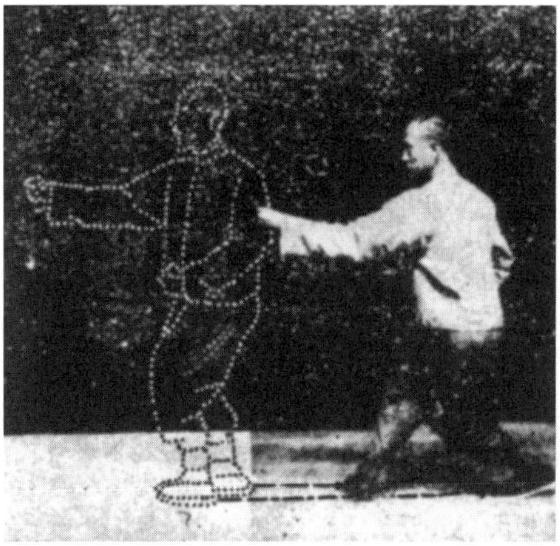

Figure 2-42.

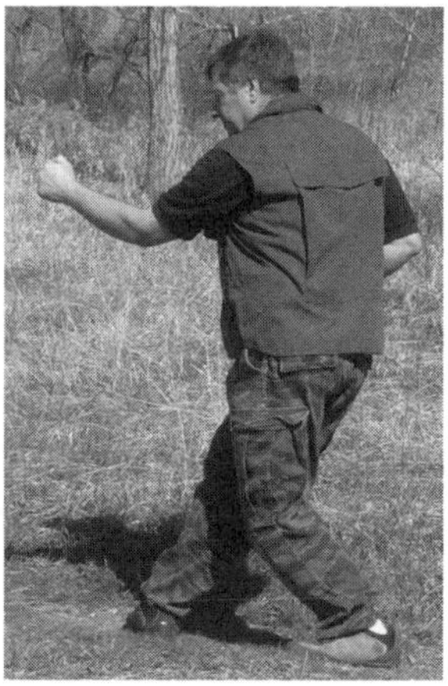

Figure 2-42m.

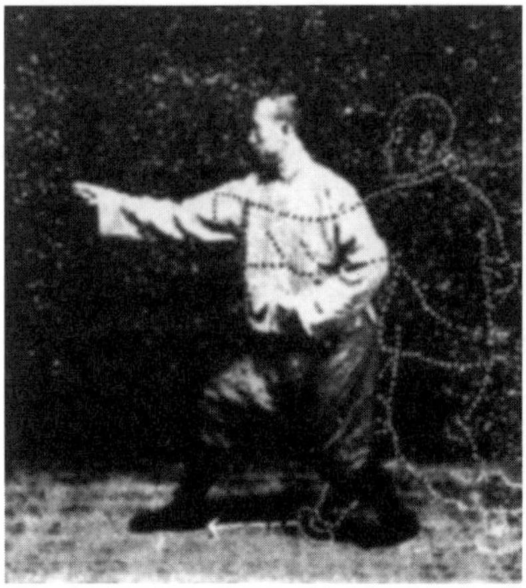

Figure 2-43.

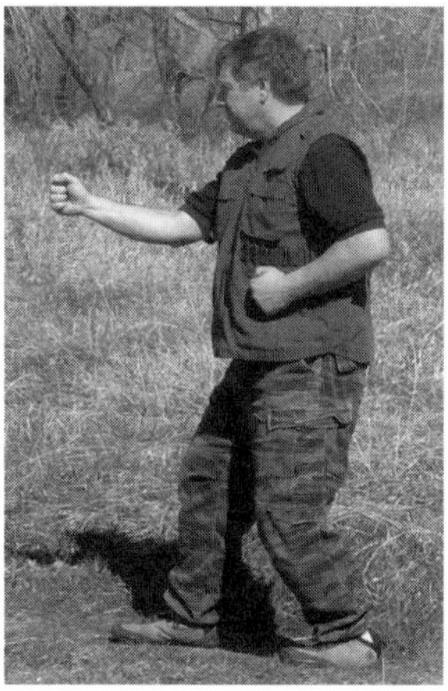

Figure 2-43m.

**Action #4** (Figures 2-44 and 2-44m1–2-44m3): Take a slight step back with the left leg. Cross both fists to form a "T" in front of the groin. Keeping their relative position, immediately raise your hands above your head. Make a half circle outward and down toward the stomach with each fist. Your right fist enters, with force, into your left palm. Raise your right leg and draw it backward toward the left leg, so legs are now close to each other. Knees are slightly bent.

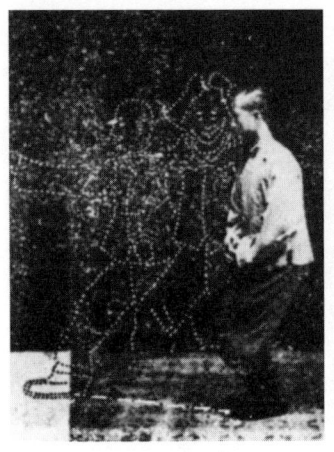

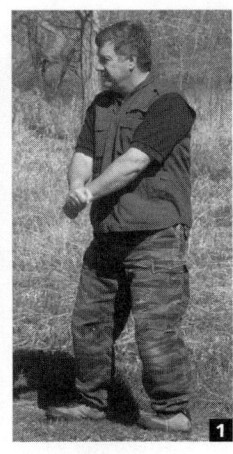

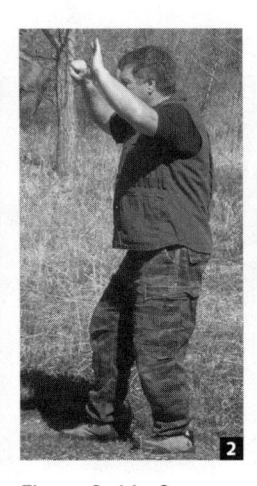

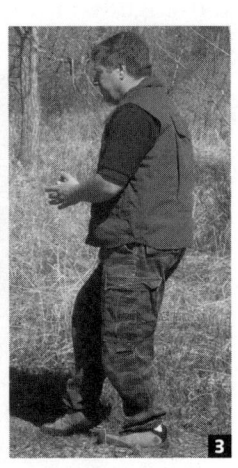

Figure 2-44.   Figure 2-44m1.   Figure 2-44m2.   Figure 2-44m3.

**Action #5** (Figures 2-45 and 2-45m): Step forward with right leg and punch straight out with left fist. As you step, align the fist with the chest. Body is forward and lead leg is slightly bent. Rear leg supports the body by pushing against the floor. Right fist flips upward and the back of the hand touches the top of the forehead. Eyes are level.

**Action #6** (Figures 2-46 and 2-46m): Make a large diagonal step backward and to the right with your right foot, so foot lands slightly behind the left leg. Right palm goes down. Punch out from the chest in a drilling movement with the left fist. Take your left foot and step back to your right foot. This results in both legs being together with knees slightly bent. Face both fists upward and place them level with the stomach. Left hand is in a horizontal position. Right hand is on top.

Figure 2-45.

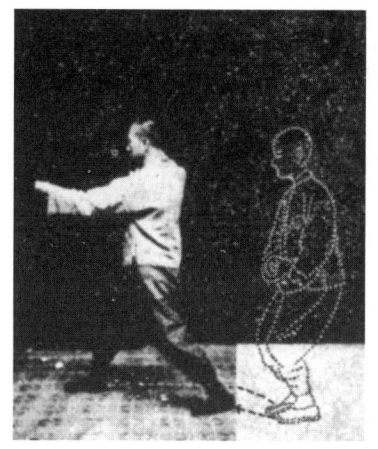

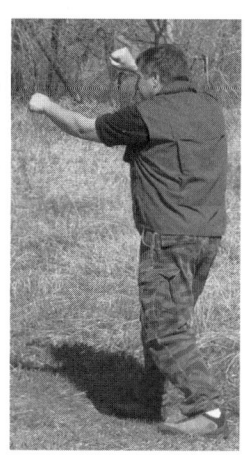

Figure 2-45m.

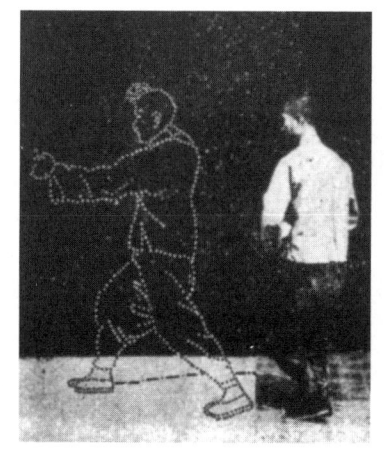

Figure 2-46.

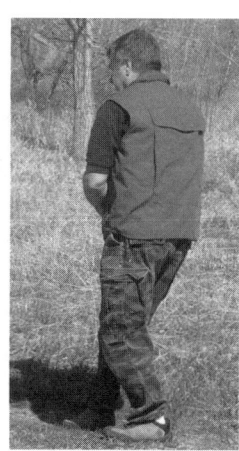

Figure 2-46m.

**Action #7** (Figures 2-47, right side of illustration, and 2-47m1): Step forward with the left leg. Swing your left palm outward and straight ahead. The back of the hand faces upward, level with the neck. Right leg and right fist retain their original position. Left leg is slightly bent. Right leg is straight. Eyes are focused on the palm in front *(focusing beyond your hand on the target)*.

**Action #8** (Figures 2-47, left side of illustration, and 2-47m2): Left leg half faces slightly forward and to the left. *(That is, you are turned slightly to the left.)* Change both palms into fists. Push the right fist out keeping the little finger facing up. Arms are slightly bent. Draw the left fist back, palm up, to the waist. Right leg is approximately one step forward. Knee is slightly bent.

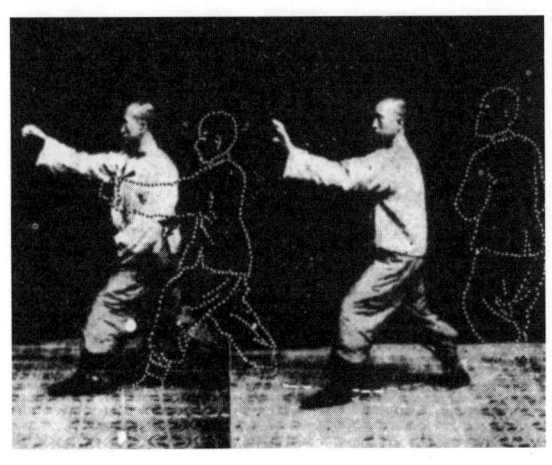

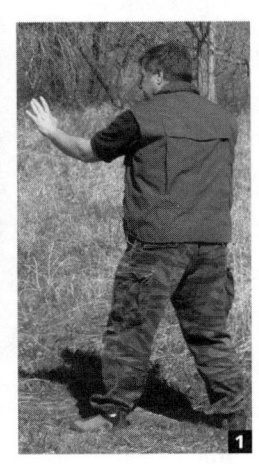

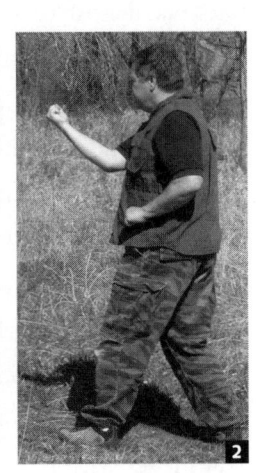

Figure 2-47.   Figure 2-47m1.   Figure 2-47m2.

**Action #9** (Figures 2-48 and 2-48m): Take a small step forward with your left foot. Turn both fists face up and keep them level with the chest. Left hand is positioned above, right hand below. Step forward with your right foot. Foot should land in a horizontally outward-turned position. Left fist turns into a palm. Turn it over and push it outward not higher than neck height. Right palm flips and pulls. Eyes are level with the palm in front. Chest is slightly forward. Front leg is slightly bent.

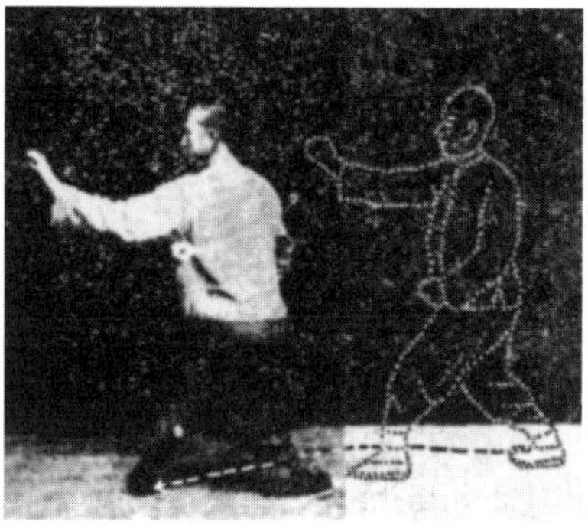

Figure 2-48.

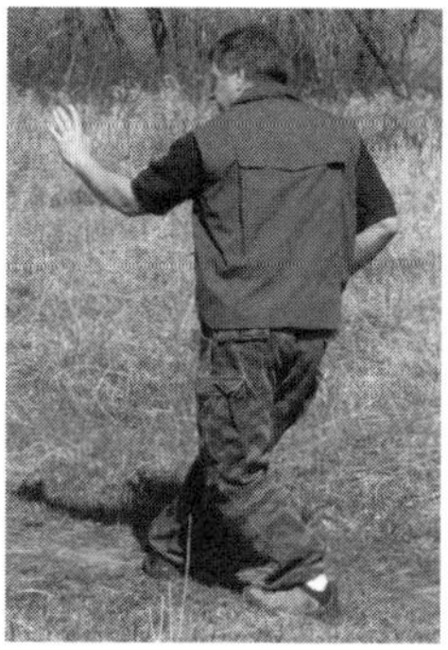

Figure 2-48m.

**Action #10** (Figures 2-49, 2-49m1, and 2-49m2): Change both hands into fists. Next, step forward with right foot. Follow this with a large step with your left foot. Immediately punch the right fist out in line with the chest. Arm is straight. As you punch, withdraw the left fist to the waist, palm facing upward. Step forward with right foot. Place your right ankle in line with the heel of your left foot. Chest is slightly forward. Slightly raise your hips. Keep both legs slightly bent.

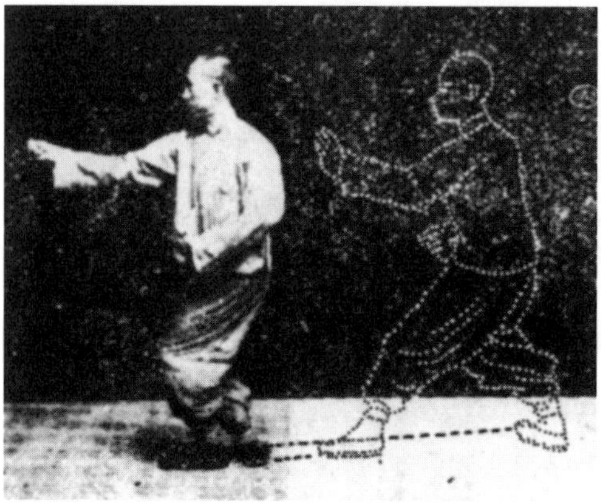

Figure 2-49.

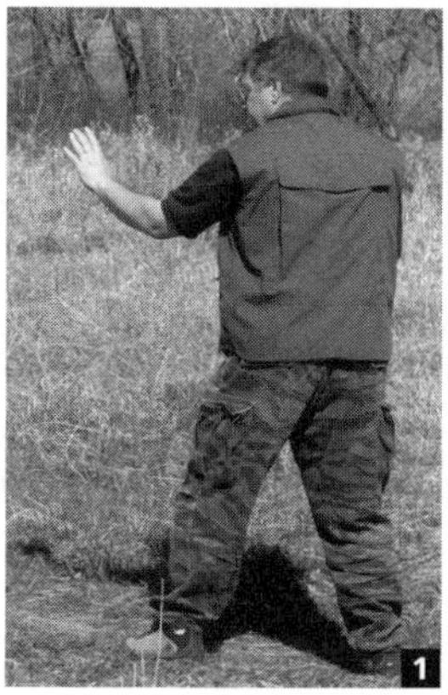

Figure 2-49m1.

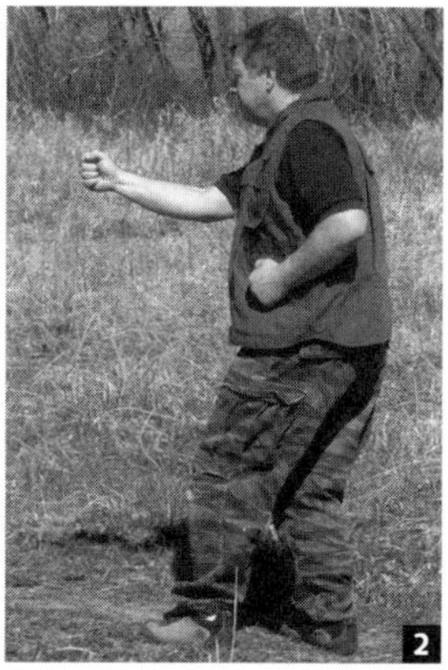

Figure 2-49m2.

## SECTION XX: TURNING AROUND IN LINKING FIST

To turn around after the tenth move, follow the orders:

*"Stop . . . to the back . . . turn."*

When you hear the order, immediately move your left foot to the right and make a right turn to the back. Lift the right foot. Use your right fist to punch out with a drilling movement. Left fist *embraces* with

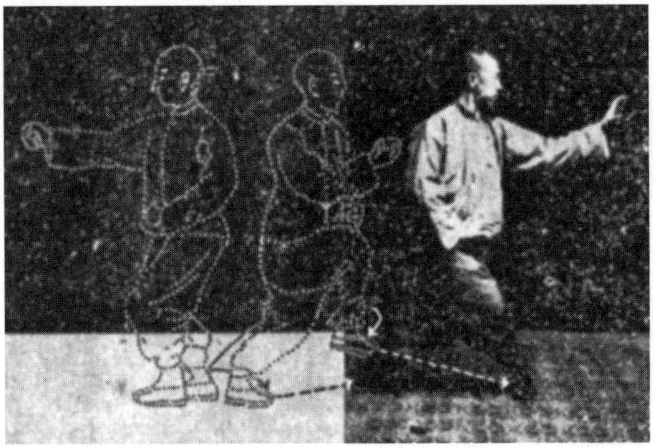

Figure 2-50.

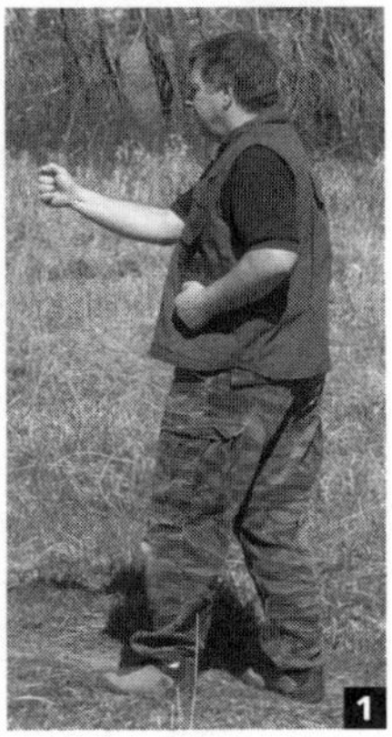

Figure 2-50m1.

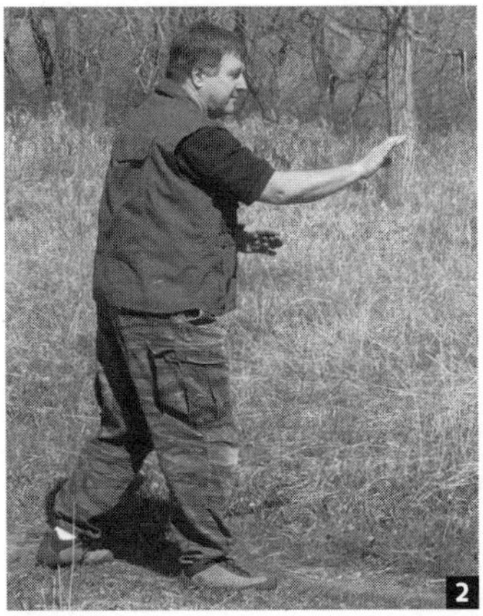

Figure 2-50m2.

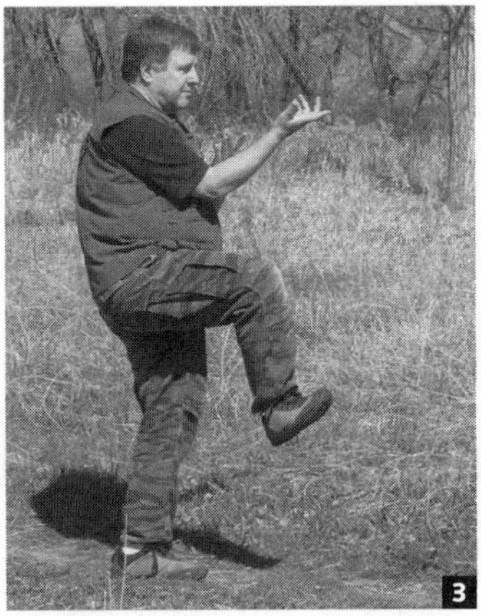

Figure 2-50m3.

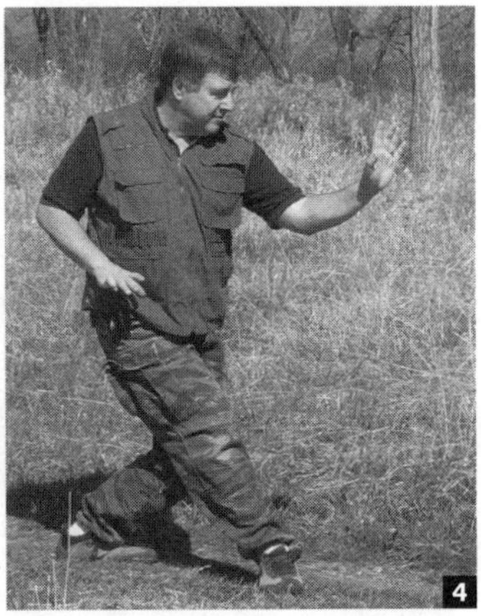

Figure 2-50m4.

the palm facing up. Immediately, push it out with force. Hand and feet land together. Both palms flip so the backs of the hands face upward. The palm at the back touches the ribs. The palm in front stretches out in front of the chest, not higher than the neck. Both arms are slightly bent.

## PICI TRAINING

Unlike the empty hand instructions in Chapter 2 of Huang's original text (which makes no mention of applications), Chapters 3 and 4 of his book clearly describe applications for each weapon technique. Also present in these sections but less obvious to the reader is Huang's outline for *pici* training.

Pici (slash/split and stab) consists of contact training and/or free sparring with wooden rifles, sabres, short weapons such as daggers or bayonets, and protective gear. Although Huang does not go into detail about conducting this type of practice, he does state that it usually occurs in stages three and four of the training process.

Figure 2-51. Illustration of pici training (ca. 1926).

Both empty hand and full contact pici training existed at the Central Military Academy at Nanjing. According to Col. Chang, development of the group took precedence over development of the individual. Training was particularly demanding and injuries were both common and acceptable. Those who fell behind in training were weeded out or, as Col. Chang bluntly stated, "they kept up or else."

The obvious reason for such a demanding approach is that survival and success in battle was predicated upon soldiers being able to "hold their own." One weak link in the chain would have resulted in failure and death of the unit.

Huang makes no mention of xingyi pici training with short weapons. This is odd for two reasons:

- Practice of this kind was well known and going on at the time of Huang's writing.
- Combat applications using dagger and bayonet are the ones most immediately identifiable with empty hand training.

While a complete study of these methods is beyond the scope of this book, they, like sabre and rifle and bayonet, are part of the logical progression from empty hand to weapons. It is for this reason I have included the two examples below.

### Armed Application #1: Splitting Fist

Your opponent attacks with a straight thrust to your chest (Figure 2-52a).

Using your bayonet, you counter with the uppercut of splitting fist (Figure 2-52b). This action deflects his rifle to the side and past your body.

Pull down and trap his weapon with the pommel of your bayonet (Figure 2-52c).

Use your palm strike to cover his weapon hand. This prevents him from escaping or striking you with the stock of your rifle (Figure 2-52d).

Counterattack with a straight thrust to his midsection or neck (Figure 2-52e).

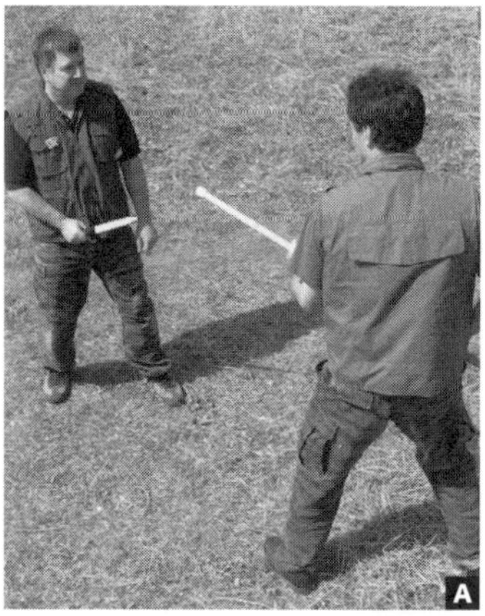

Chapter Two    **57**

Figure 2-52a.

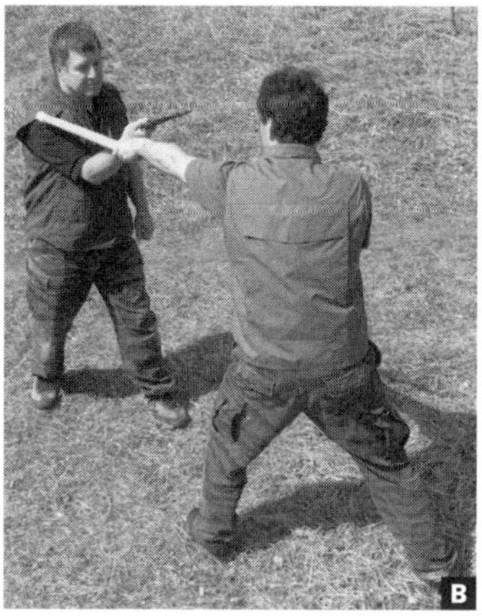

Figure 2-52b.

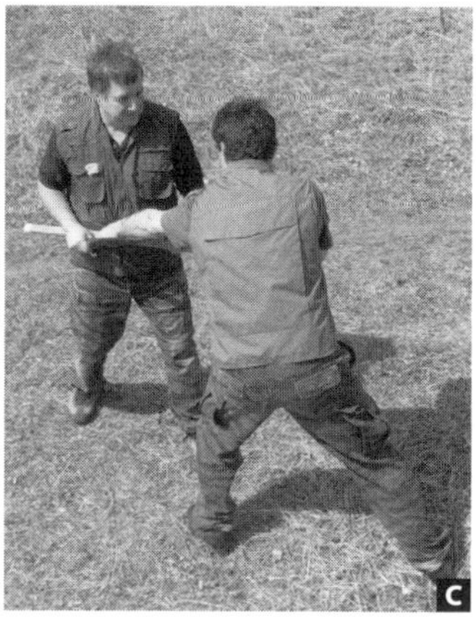

Figure 2-52c.

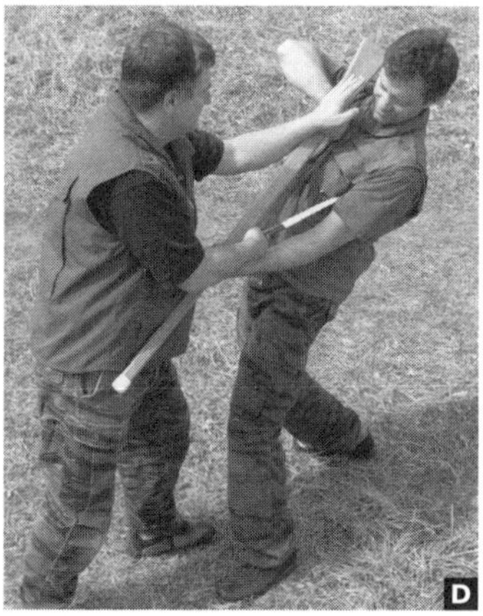

Figure 2-52d.

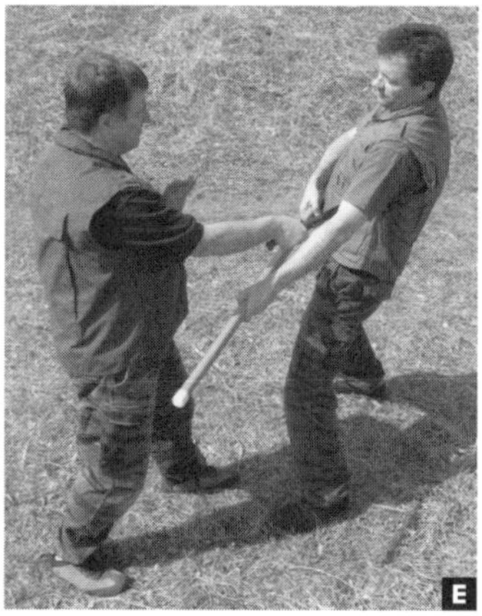

Figure 2-52e.

## Armed Application #2: Pounding Fist

Here your opponent attacks the left side of your upper body (Figure 2-53a).

Use the blocking and stepping action of pounding fist to deflect and grab his weapon (Figure 2-53b).

Counter with a straight thrust to his exposed side (Figure 2-53c).

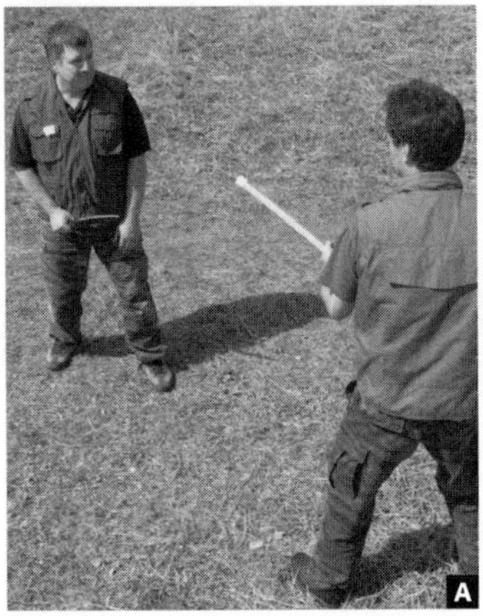

Figure 2-53a.

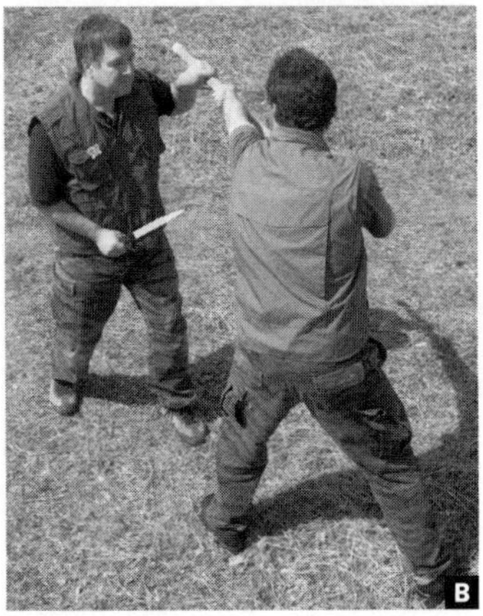

Figure 2-53b.

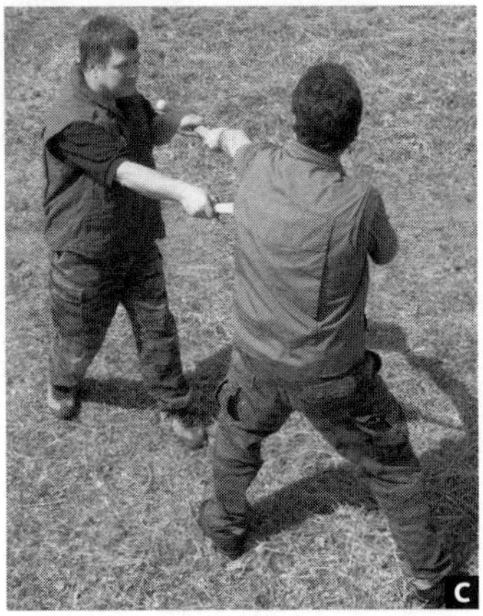

Figure 2-53c.

## Incorrect Instinctive Response

Because of the fear of being cut, most of us will attempt to keep the bayonet away from our face (Figure 2-54a). Such a reaction results in the loss of mechanical advantage. The opponent simply pulls his weapon back and realigns it with his body (Figure 2-54b)—ready to attack again (Figure 2-54c).

Proper blocking and seizing dictates that you pull the weapon near your head while keeping your elbows down (Figure 2-54d). This gives you superiority of leverage and allows complete control of his movement.

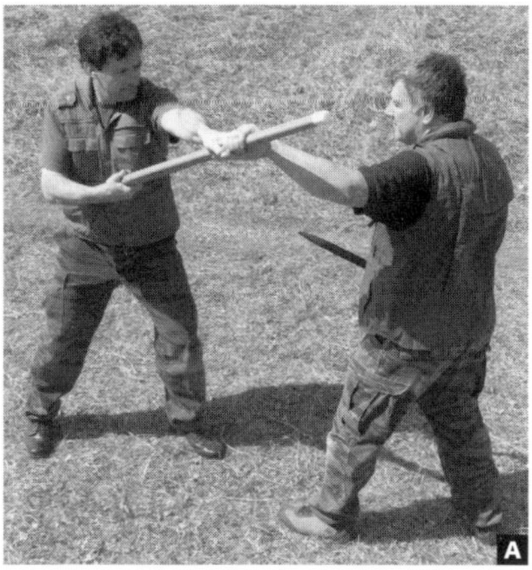

Chapter Two 59

Figure 2-54a.

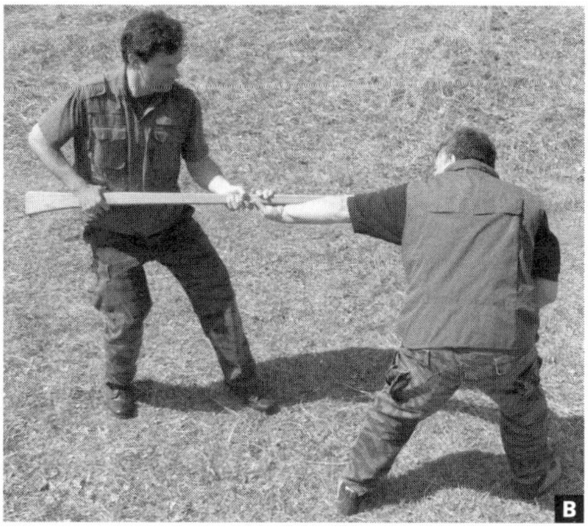

Figure 2-54b.

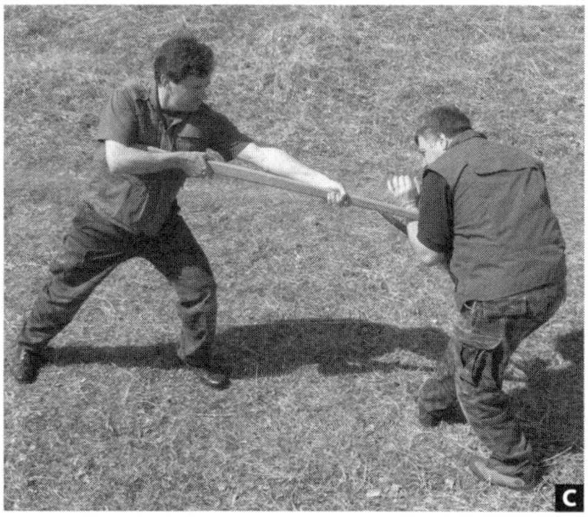

Figure 2-54c.

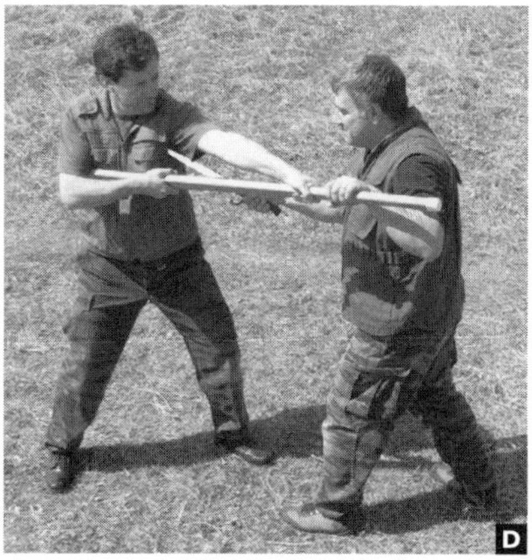

Figure 2-54d.

# Chapter 3

# SECTION I: RIFLE AND BAYONET TRAINING

Xingyi rifle and bayonet training is divided into two major sections. Section one involves training with a real rifle and bayonet. Its primary goal is to train the wrist for actual confrontation. Section two employs a wooden rifle in training. This helps determine ability. Both sections are further broken down into four categories:

Thrusting (*defending and attacking*)

Floating or flowing—continuous action and combination techniques

Two-person exercises (*prearranged sparring*)

No pattern (*freestyle fighting*)

In category one, thrusting is only used to make forward *(attacking)* movements. No backward *(retreating)* movements are employed. The purpose of this is to instill the goal of killing the enemy.

Category two employs both advancing [forward] and withdrawing [backward] movements. Here the idea is to link the individual techniques into patterns of continuous motion. This result denies the enemy an opportunity to retaliate.

In practicing the two-person exercises of category three, the wooden rifle is used. Exercises are performed back and forth to develop hand-eye coordination. Practitioners are only allowed to follow prearranged patterns.

Category four also utilizes the wooden rifle and two men fighting against each other. This training is freestyle, utilizing movement in no fixed order. Combatants, wearing masks for protection, fight using their imagination and all they have been taught. Performance is scored and evaluated.

To make it easier to teach these methods, actions and applications are combined. One reason for this is it makes it easy to understand. Another reason is that we hope to get people interested *(in training)*. We imagine our opponent attacking us from a certain position so that we are able to standardize this series of exercises.

## HOLDING RIFLE AND STANDING AT ATTENTION

Figure 3-1 illustrates *standing at attention*. To change from *holding rifle position* to *attention position*, respond to the order:

*"Attention."*

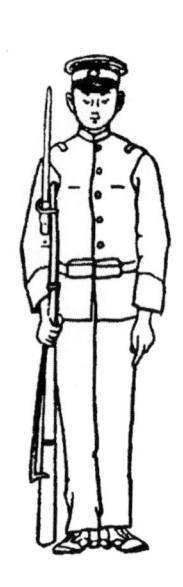

Figure 3-1.

## READY POSITION

To make the transition from standing at attention to *ready position*, follow the orders:

*"Ready . . . with rifle . . . thrust."*

**Action #1:** Stand with the left foot and head pointing straight ahead. Angle the body slightly to the right.

**Action #2** (Figure 3-2): Using the right hand, lift the rifle to a position where the hand is level with the shoulder. Rifle barrel remains vertical and the weapon moves along the right side of the body. At the same time, use your left hand to grasp the stock. Both elbows touch the ribs.

Figure 3-2.    Figure 3-3.    Figure 3-4.

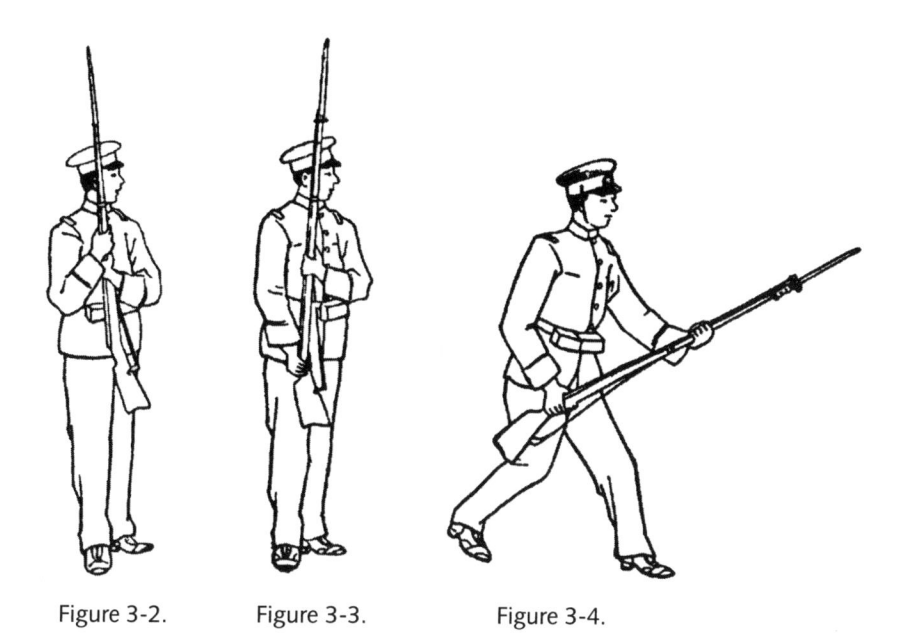

**Action #3** (Figure 3-3): Move your right arm vertically down the rifle. Lightly grasp the stock behind the trigger well with your right hand.

**Action #4** (Figure 3-4): Take a half-step forward with your left foot. Knees are slightly bent and the weight of the body is evenly distributed between the two feet. As this action occurs, push the weapon forward with both hands.

Point the *face* of the weapon upward and position your right hand on the right side of the stomach. Slightly bend your elbow. The lower section of the rifle is held on a horizontal level. Bayonet points to the opponent's eyes. *(The actual angle of the rifle is approximately 15 degrees from horizontal.)* Body pose is natural with weight centered and eyes fixed upon the enemy.

*(Note: It is important you assume the ready position by stepping forward instead of backward. The forward movement trains you to close distance when performing both offensive and defensive tactics.*

*All exercises, whether solo or against an opponent, begin with soldiers standing at attention and then moving into the ready position.)*

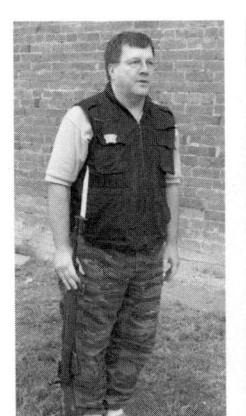

Figure 3-5a. Stand at attention.

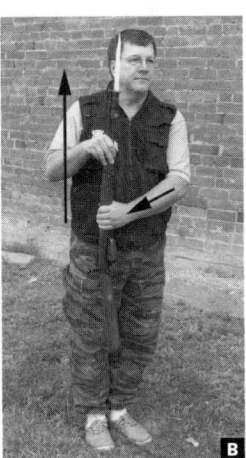

Figure 3-5b. Lift the rifle and grasp the stock.

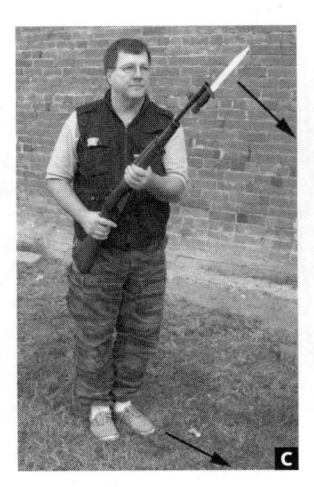

Figure 3-5c. Drop the rifle point as you step forward with your left foot.

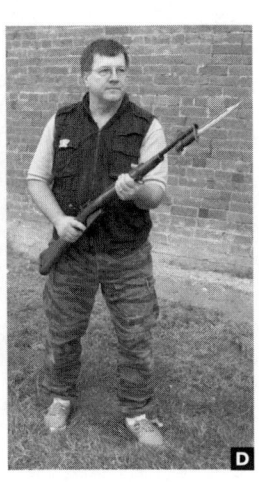

Figure 3-5d. Use the rifle to cover your body.

## EXPLANATION OF THRUSTING

### Reinforcing Step

The basic rifle and bayonet thrust in xingyi uses a reinforcing step. Here the rifle thrust is performed after the lead foot steps and coincides with the reinforcing action of the rear foot. That is, thrust as you move and plant your rear foot.

The break in timing between moving your front foot and thrusting is vital for the success of the attack. If you thrust as your lead foot steps, your body performs a gross motor movement that is easily seen (and blocked!) by your opponent. By stepping first, then thrusting, you break the timing of your attack. This change in timing confuses your opponent and reduces his ability to parry your attack.

Additionally, coupling your attack with the reinforcing action of your rear foot dramatically increases the force of your thrust. The weight and momentum of your body combines with the action of your thrust to produce a force that is greater than the force generated by your arms alone.

## No Lunge

Western-style bayonet fighting theory traditionally teaches soldiers to lunge when executing either long or short thrusts. Often, to gain greater reach, the heel of the rear foot will even leave the ground. Resembling a fencer's lunge, this technique does enable the soldier to obtain a good reach. Its downfall, however, lies in the fact that unlike sport fencing, close combat does not occur on a dry, flat surface. Field conditions in war are less than ideal. Controlled attack and recovery in real-life settings (mud, gravel, deep brush, ice, debris, etc.) become extremely difficult from a deep lunge position. (In order to prepare their soldiers, the People's Liberation Army [PLA] still practice bayonet sparring on uneven terrain, elevated narrow bridges, and in all sorts of weather and ground conditions.)

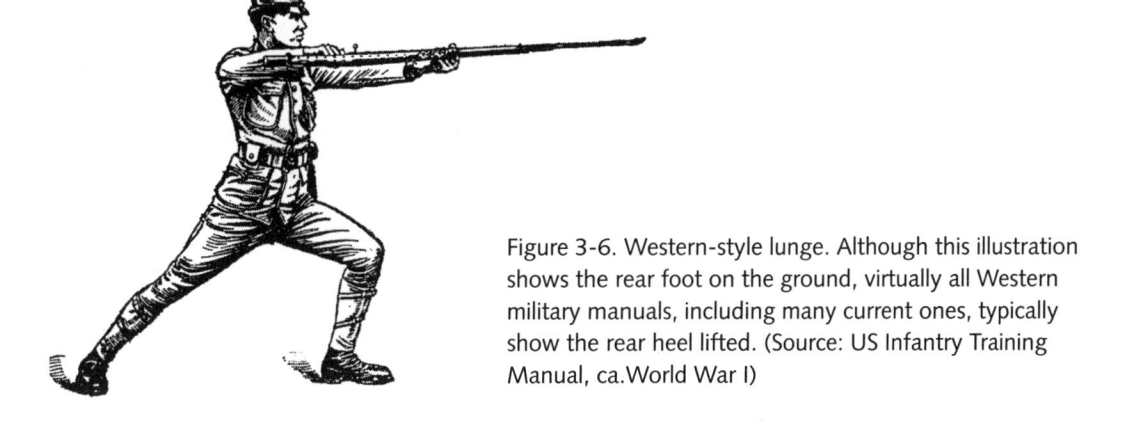

Figure 3-6. Western-style lunge. Although this illustration shows the rear foot on the ground, virtually all Western military manuals, including many current ones, typically show the rear heel lifted. (Source: US Infantry Training Manual, ca. World War I)

In contrast, xingyi rifle and bayonet methods have no lunge. Armed xingyi exponents always use the reinforcing step when thrusting. Such movement accomplishes at least three goals:

- It provides stability and maneuverability (thus, no problem in recovering balance or moving).
- It avoids the overextension and resulting exposure created by the deep lunge.
- It assists in disrupting the enemy's range of attack.

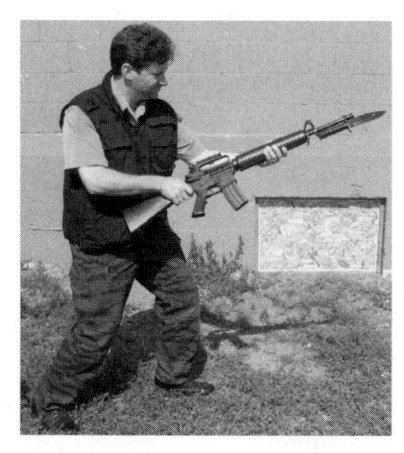

Figure 3-7. Xingyi reinforcing step, with no lunge.

## Rolling the Wrist

When performing either blocks or short thrusts, xingyi emphasizes rolling the wrist of the lead hand—an action similar to the fist rotation in drilling. Rolling the hand in this manner increases your leverage by bringing your elbows closer to your body (Figure 3-8). This in turn can be used to control the movement and position of your opponent's weapon.

Rolling the wrist and maintaining contact allows you to feel the attacker's movement. You can control his movement, slide down his barrel, and easily cut his lead hand (Figure 3-9).

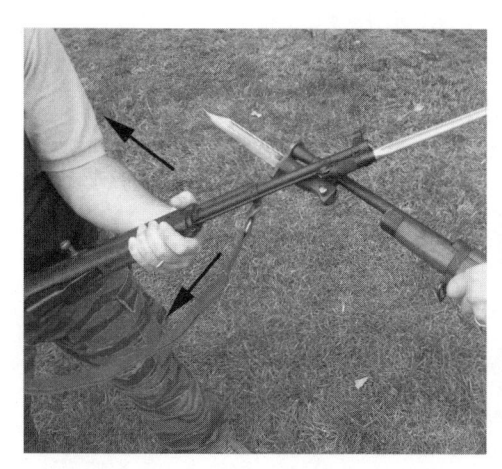

Figure 3-8.

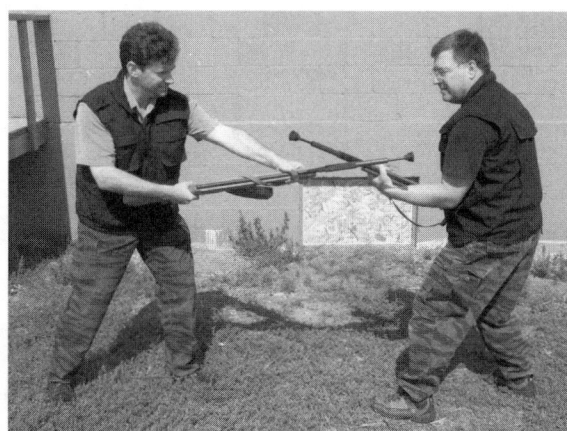

Figure 3-9.

In contrast, the Western trained exponent of bayonet fighting is simply taught to knock the enemy's weapon out of the way and execute a counterattack before the enemy has an opportunity to recover.

While knocking does move the enemy's weapon out of the way, it does not control his ability to recover prior to your counterattack. (Knocking also prevents you from feeling your opponent's reaction.) In xingyi, weapons contact and tend to remain in contact. This allows you to accurately gauge your opponent's movement or resistance—much in the same manner as the *tui shou* (pushing hands) exercise of *tai ji quan*.

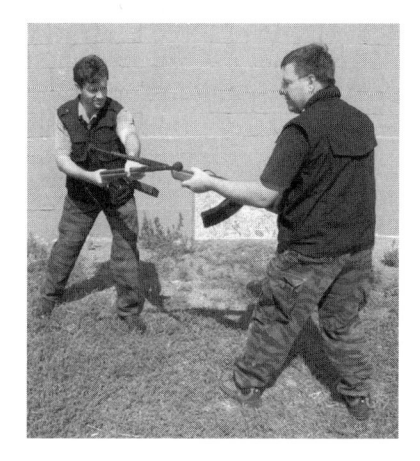

Figure 3-10. Here the defender knocks the attacker's weapon aside.

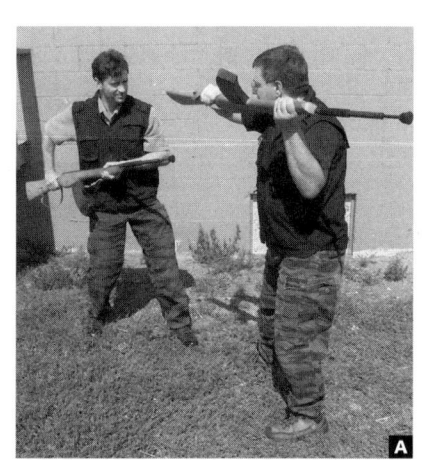

Figure 3-11a. To deliver a butt stroke, the defender breaks contact with his attacker's weapon. This allows the attacker to retract his rifle.

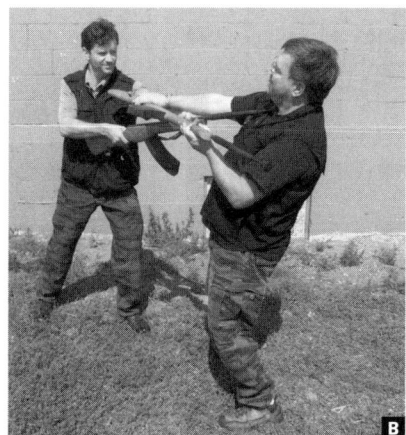

Figure 3-11b. The attacker can then counterattack with a straight thrust.

## THRUSTING I

To make the transition from ready position to *thrusting position*, follow the command:

*"Thrust."*

**Action #1** (Figure 3-12): Imagine that your opponent is thrusting to your face. Immediately roll your left hand and wrist. Lead hand points to the mouth. Your arms rest on the chest. Your back hand touches the right hip. As you roll the wrist, lean forward slightly so that your left shoulder and bayonet are aligned. Immediately stamp the right foot and execute a counterthrust to the opponent's throat.

**Action #2** (Figure 3-12): Begin by holding the rifle tightly (and without movement) against the upper body. Stamp hard with the right foot to assist the left foot in traveling forward. Distance covered should be approximately 2 feet. Right leg remains slightly bent, forming *step thrust position*.

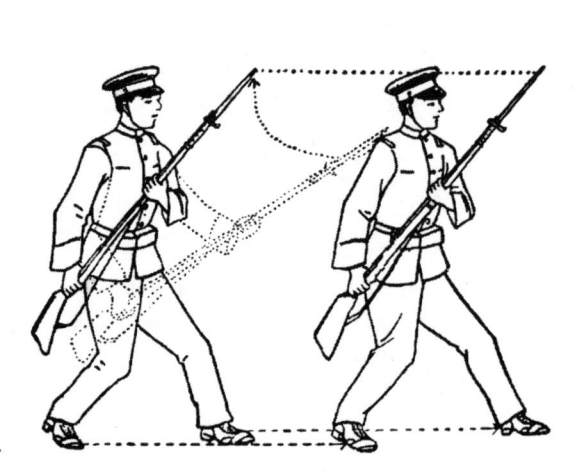

Figure 3-12.

## EXPLANATION OF BODY ALIGNMENT

Besides proper stance, your rifle and bayonet must be positioned in such a manner as to cover or protect your center line. This reduces your opponent's targets because his thrust must occur on either the right or left edge of your body. Additionally, since his line of attack to vital parts of your body is now an indirect attack, around your rifle, this makes it easier for you to block.

## DRILLS FOR THRUSTING I
### One- or Two-Person Drill

This drill combines Actions #1 and #2. Action #1 and #2 can be done separately (as described by Huang) or they can be combined together against either an imaginary opponent (solo drill) or real opponent (two-person exercise). As a solo drill, Actions #1 and #2 can be combined and performed in the following manner:

Execute the block and counterthrust (with reinforcing step forward) as described in Action #1.

Immediately after you thrust, retract your weapon and return to the ready position.

Repeat the block and counterthrust. Retract your weapon as you move forward.

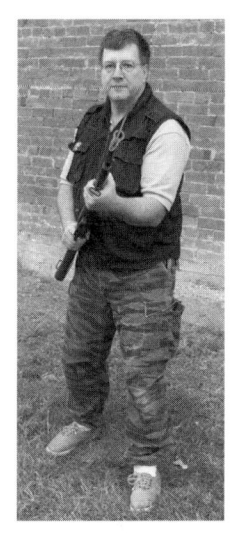

Figure 3-13.

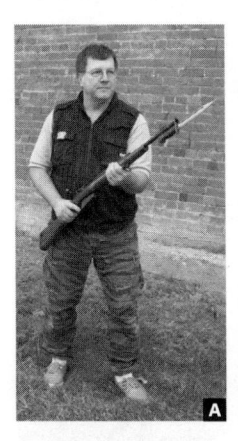

Figure 3-14a. Begin from ready position.

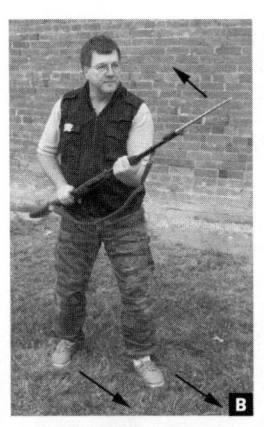

Figure 3-14b. Execute the block by rolling your wrists as you take a reinforcing step forward.

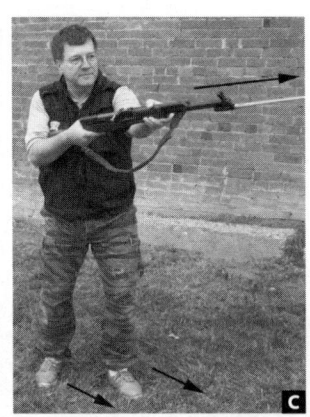

Figure 3-14c. Step forward again and deliver a straight thrust.

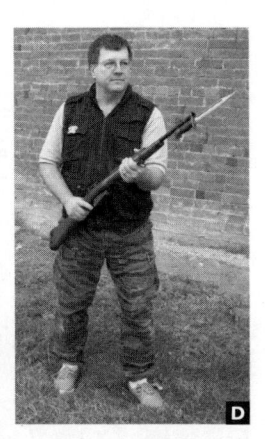

Figure 3-14d. Return to the ready position and repeat the sequence. Alternately, shift stance and practice the sequence with your right foot forward.

## Two-Person Drill: Block/Thrust (Fixed Position)

Face your opponent while standing at attention.

When the instructor gives the verbal signal "ready," assume a left-foot-forward *san ti shi,* or trinity stance. Continue to face each other and make sure that you are both slightly out of each other's range of attack.

On a verbal signal from your instructor, your opponent attacks with a straight thrust to the left side of your chest.

Counter by rolling both wrists. Draw the stock of your rifle back so that your right hand rests on your right side, by your hip. Use the barrel of your rifle and bayonet to deflect his weapon and carry it past you on your left side.

Keep your barrel and bayonet pointed to the front, facing your opponent.

Immediately follow the deflection with a counterattack. Remember to reinforce the step and thrust as you plant your rear foot.

Step back to the starting position and repeat this attack and counter sequence for a set number of repetitions.

After the set is completed, reverse rolls. You become the attacker while your partner defends and counters.

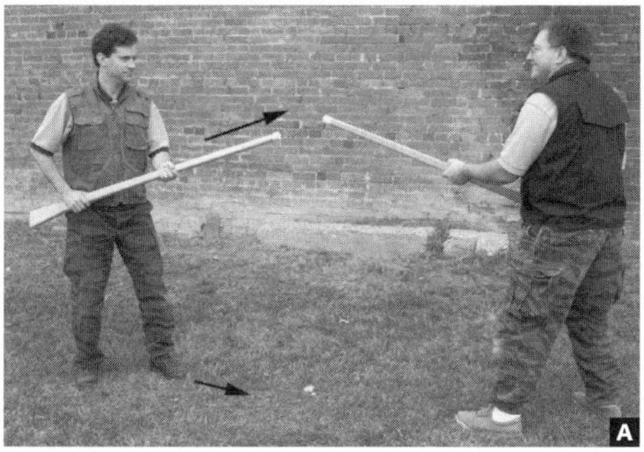

Figure 3-15a. Opponent attacks with a straight thrust to your left side.

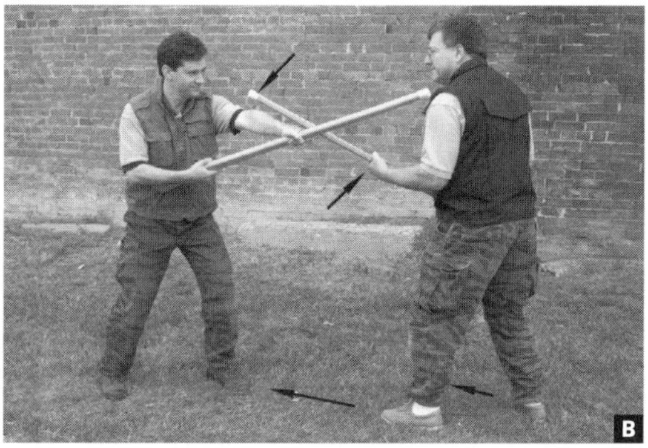

Figure 3-15b. You block by rolling both wrists and closing distance. Stepping puts you inside his range of attack.

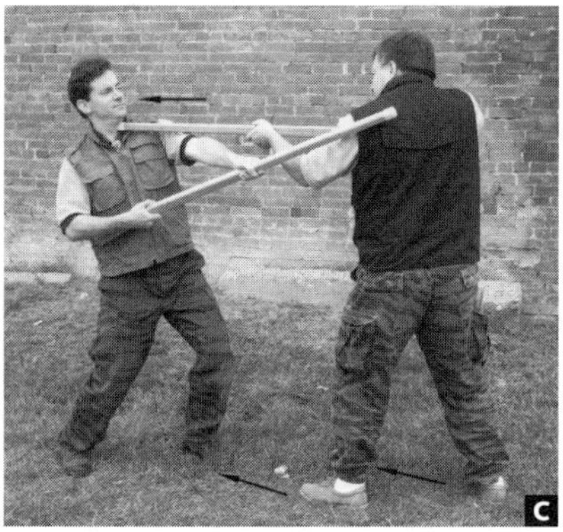

Figure 3-15c. Counter with a straight thrust to his upper body.

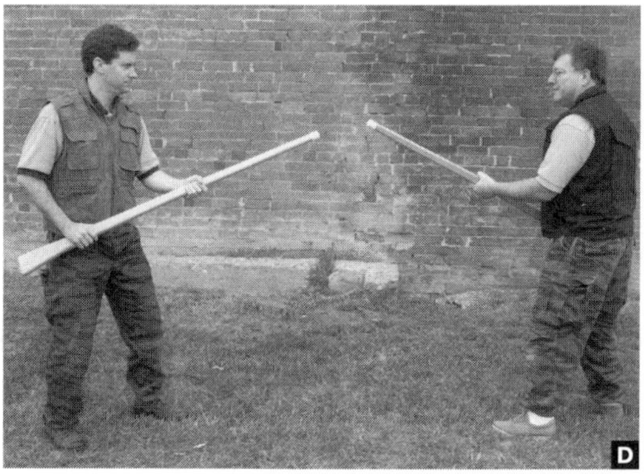

Figure 3-15d. Step back into the ready position and repeat the exercise.

There are several variations of this two-person drill. They increase in complexity as the skill of the practitioners improves. Two variations of the basic drill, in which attacks and counterattacks alternate as a back-and-forth exercise, are explained below.

## Variation #1: Alternating Attack and Defense (Fixed Position)

Your opponent attacks with a thrust.

You block, take a reinforcing step forward, and counterattack.

Your opponent immediately withdraws. He quickly blocks and uses a reinforcing step forward to counterattack.

You withdraw, block, and counterattack.

Repeat these back-and-forth actions for a set number of repetitions.

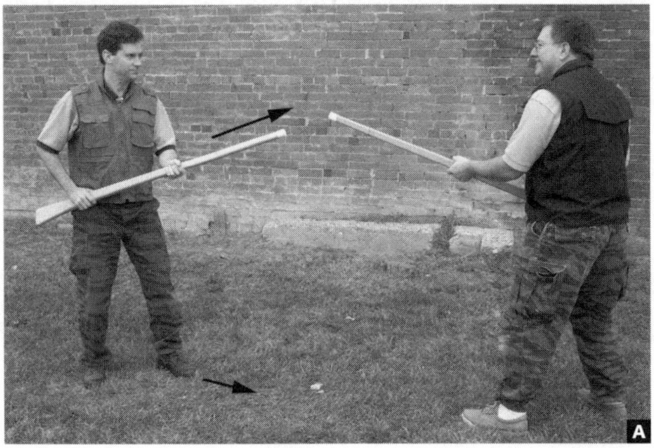

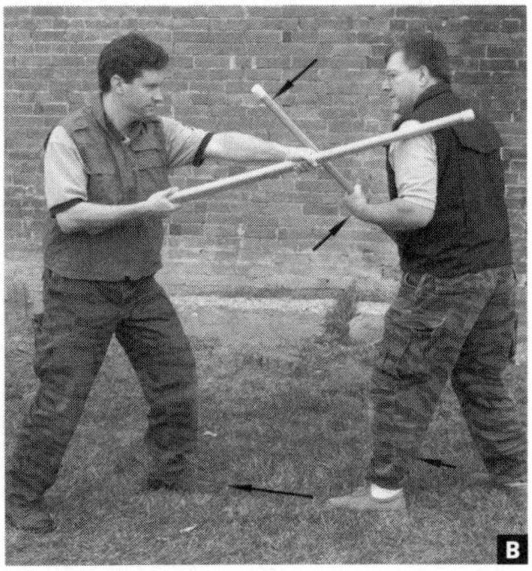

Figure 3-16a. Opponent attacks with a straight thrust to your upper left side.

Figure 3-16b. Block and move inside his range of attack.

Chapter Three 73

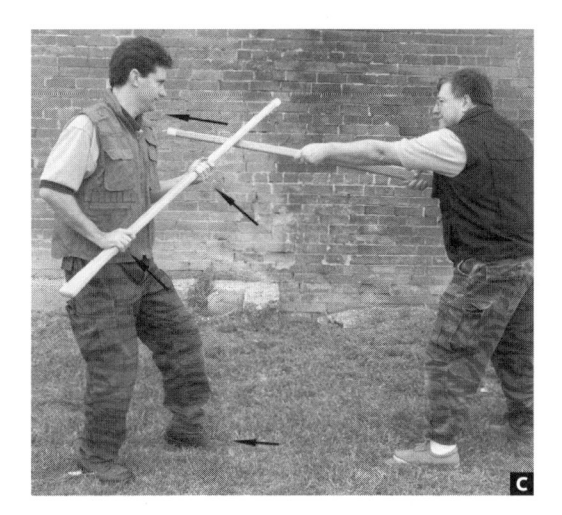

Figure 3-16c. He blocks and withdraws.

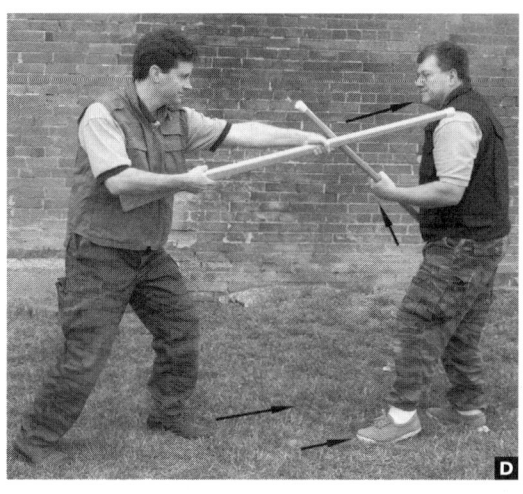

Figure 3-16d. As he counterattacks, you withdraw and block.

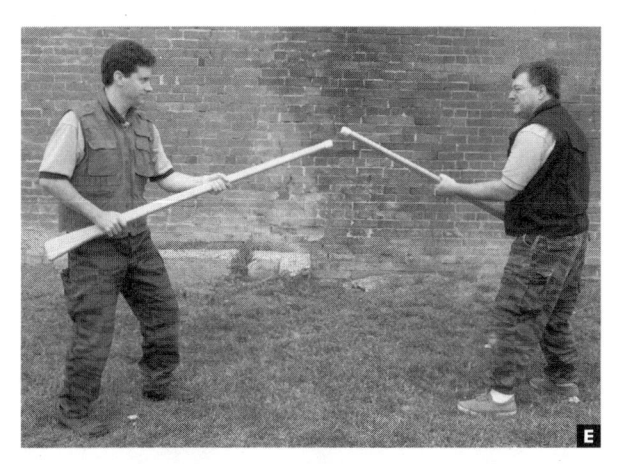

Figure 3-16e. Return to the start position. Repeat back-and-forth attack and defense actions as you vary the timing.

## Variation #2: Linear Movement

Your opponent attacks with a straight thrust.

You block, step forward, and counterthrust.

Your opponent steps back and repeats the attack as you continue to move forward, counterattacking after every block.

Once you and your partner-opponent have traversed a designated length (e.g., 50 feet), reverse roles. That is, your opponent defends while you attack.

Repeat for a set number of repetitions.

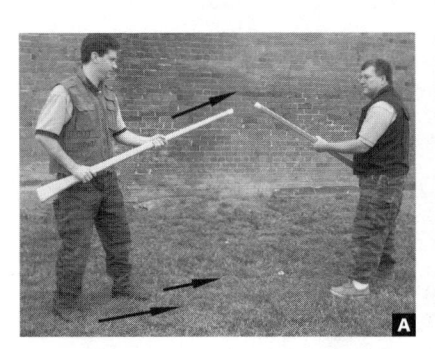

Figure 3-17a. Your opponent attacks with a straight thrust.

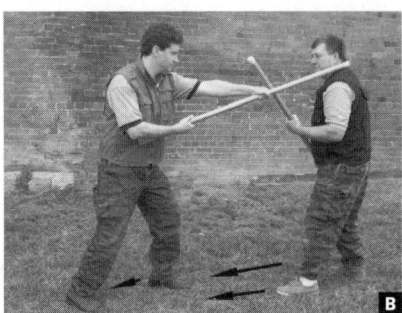

Figure 3-17b. You block, step forward, and counterattack with a straight thrust.

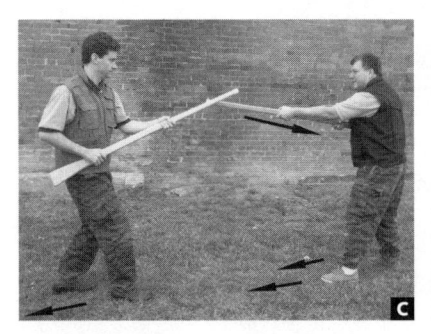

Figure 3-17c. Your opponent steps back with his lead foot. He quickly follows this by stepping back again with his rear foot. (You withdraw your rifle and prepare for another attack.)

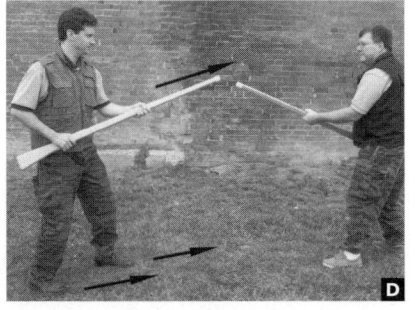

Figure 3-17d. Your opponent repeats his thrust attack.

Chapter Three 75

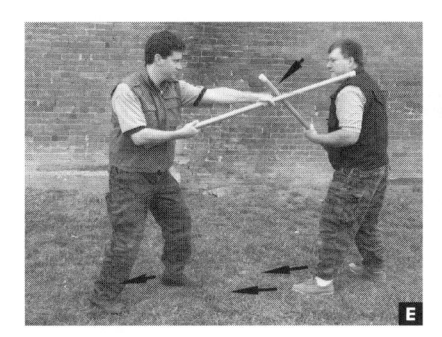

Figure 3-17e. You block and close distance to counter. (Note: in actual combat you can slash his lead hand.)

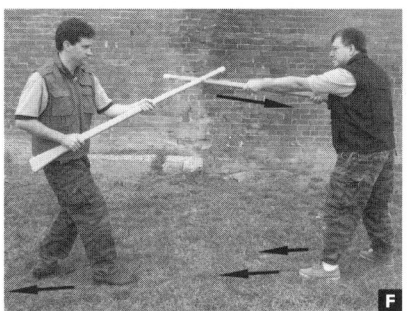

Figure 3-17f. He again steps back and prepares to attack again.

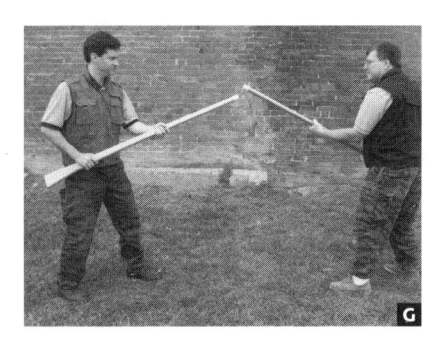

Figure 3-17g. Reverse roles and perform the exercise in the opposite direction.

## Alternative Target Areas in Actual Combat

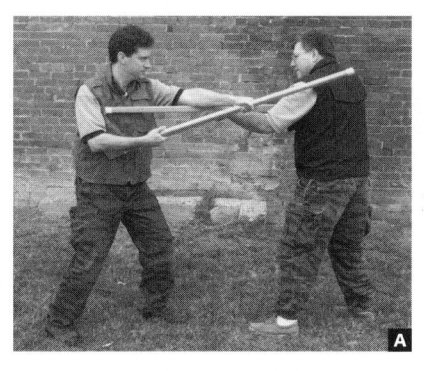

Figure 3-18a. Slip under the lead arm. Strike the chest or shoulder joints.

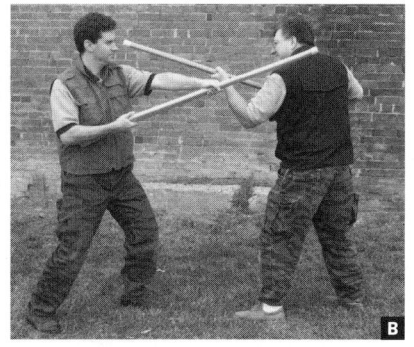

Figure 3-18b. Block and execute a horizontal slash to opponent's face.

## THRUSTING II

**Action #3** (Figure 3-19): Your opponent thrusts at your chest. Immediately roll both wrists upright so rifle and bayonet assume a *horizontal blade position. (The blade of the bayonet is flat, not vertical.)* Next, make a circular movement [loop] to the right. This deflects the opponent's weapon to the front right position. Simultaneously move the right foot forward. *(The illustration shows a scissor step to close distance.)* Land your foot hard and assume a *horizontal position (foot turned outward)*.

**Action #4** (Figure 3-20): Left foot is forward. Draw your right foot up one-half step so both feet are almost side by side. Use both hands to hold the rifle. Thrust the bayonet into your opponent's stomach. This is known as the *crushing rifle position*.

*(The looping actions described and illustrated in Action #3 and Action #4 refer to the previously mentioned rolling of the wrist when blocking and thrusting.)*

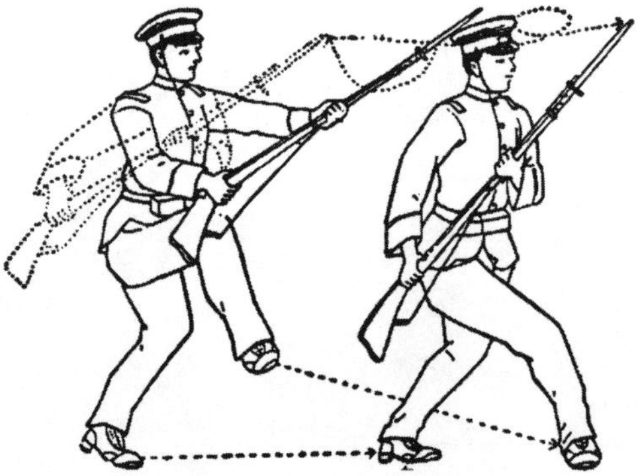

Figure 3-19.

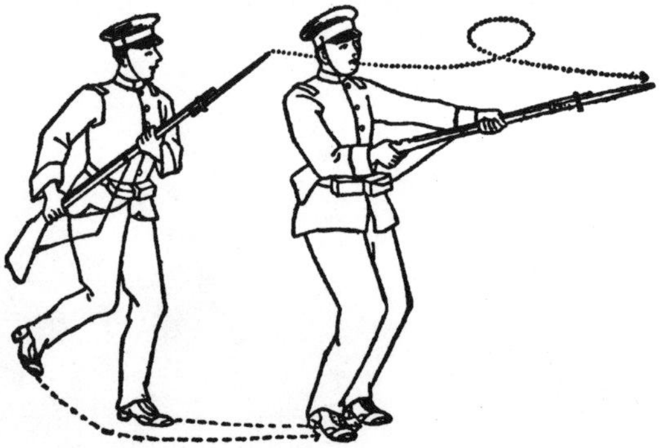

Figure 3-20.

# DRILLS FOR THRUSTING II
## Two-Person Drill: Block/Thrust with Cross-Step

Stand at attention and face your opponent.

When the instructor gives the verbal signal "ready," assume a left-foot-forward san ti stance. Continue to face each other and make sure that you are both slightly out of each other's range of attack.

On a verbal signal from the instructor, your partner attacks with a straight thrust to the right side of your chest.

Counter by rolling both wrists and drawing the rifle back so that your right hand rests on your right side, by your hip. Couple this movement with your hip action, and turn to the right to deflect his weapon to your front right position. Remember to keep your weapon pointed in the direction of your opponent.

As you block, cross-step forward with your right (rear) foot and plant it in front. Immediately step through with your left foot and thrust.

Your opponent immediately moves backward and prepares for another attack. Continue to move forward down the practice area.

Once you have moved the length of the practice area, reverse roles. Continue back and forth along the length of the practice area for an agreed-upon number of repetitions.

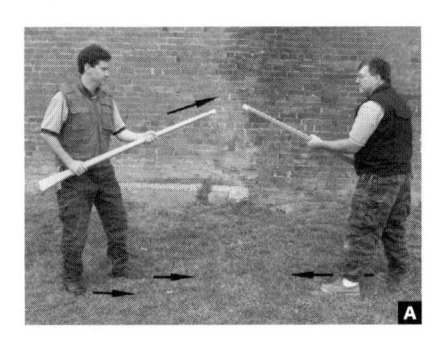

Figure 3-21a. Your opponent attacks the right side of your chest.

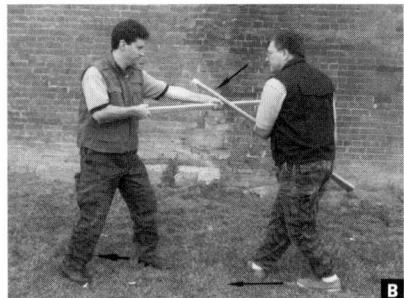

Figure 3-21b. Counter by cross-stepping, rolling your wrist, and turning to the right.

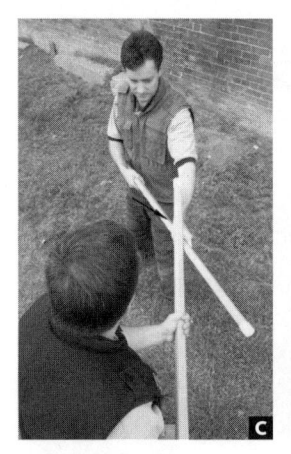

Figure 3-21c. Drop your weight onto the opponent's rifle.

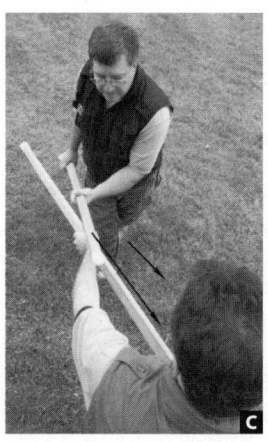

Figure 3-21c. Reverse view.

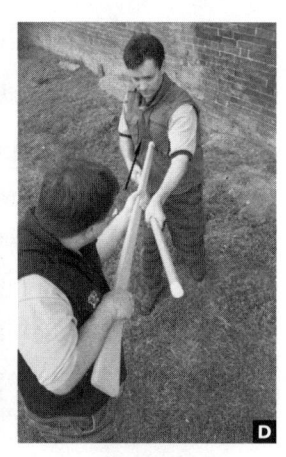

Figure 3-21d. Step through and thrust.

From this point in the exercise, you can return to the start position and either repeat the exercise in place or reverse roles.

For the purposes of this text, we will continue the exercise as a two-person linear movement drill, as previously described.

After returning to the ready position, either repeat the drill or reverse directions.

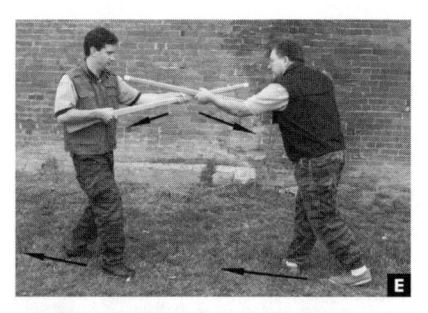

Figure 3-21e. Your opponent first cross-steps back with his lead foot. As you close distance and thrust, he takes another step back with the opposite foot. You both withdraw your weapons.

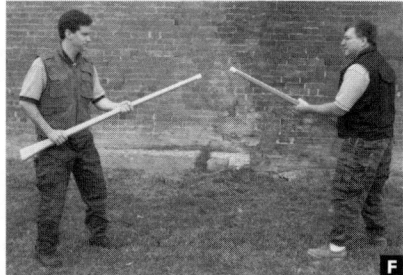

Figure 3-21f. Return to the ready position.

## APPLICATION OF THRUSTING I AND THRUSTING II

Both Thrusting I (Actions #1 and #2) and Thrusting II (Actions #3 and #4) are defense and counterattacks against a straight thrust to your chest.

In Thrusting I, the attack is aimed at your left side.

Deflect the attack by rolling your wrist, and lean forward to align your bayonet with your left shoulder. This action carries the attacker's blade past your body.

Once you have redirected the attack, maintain contact with his rifle and step forward to move inside the range of his bayonet blade.

Couple your counterthrust with the reinforcing step of your rear foot.

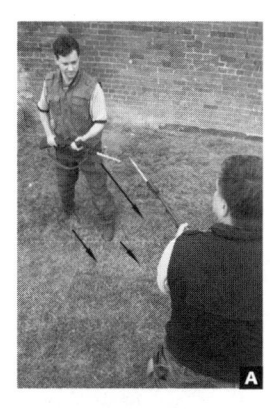

Figure 3-22a. Your opponent attacks with a straight thrust or slash to your left side.

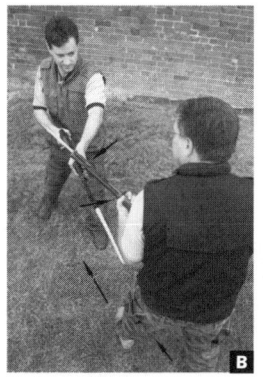

Figure 3-22b. You redirect the attack by rolling your wrists and turning your body or rifle to your left. You immediately step in to close distance and move inside your opponent's range of attack.

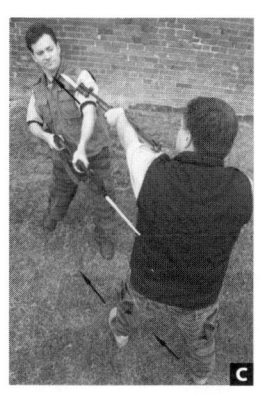

Figure 3-22c. Counterattack with a straight thrust to your opponent's near side of the body.

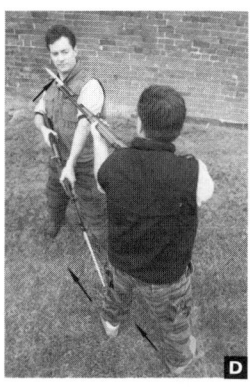

Figure 3-22d. Or slash the opponent's face.

In Thrusting II, your opponent is attacking the right side of your chest. Counter by using the same wrist rolling action as in Thrusting I.

As you roll your wrist, turn your body to the right in order to redirect the attack past your right side.

Maintain contact with your opponent's rifle.

Keep your body straight and cross-step to close distance. Note: To create a powerful counter, you must combine your cross-step and wrist rolling action. This causes the weight of your body to drop onto your opponent's rifle. The cleaver-like action can easily be directed against his lead hand (holding the stock and barrel of the rifle). This force can easily cut, sever, or break his hand or fingers. At the very least, your blow will cause him to release his grip and prevent him from parrying your attack.

Deliver a counterthrust into his midsection.

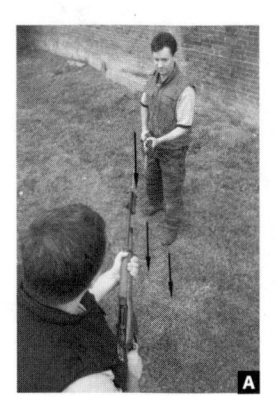

Figure 3-23a. Your opponent attacks the upper right side of your body.

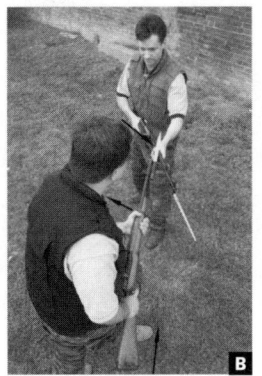

Figure 3-23b. You counter by rolling your wrist and turning your body and rifle to the right. As you cross-step to close distance, drop the weight of your body and rifle down onto your opponent's weapon.

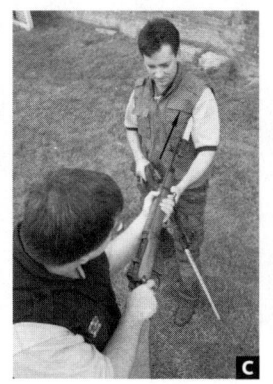

Figure 3-23c. Counter-attack with a straight thrust to the opponent's upper body or shoulder joint.

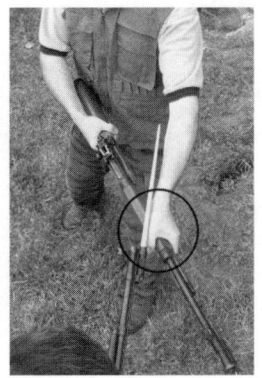

Figure 3-24. The cleaver-like action is directed against the opponent's lead hand (holding the stock and barrel of the rifle).

## JOINT ATTACKS

Another xingyi bayonet tactic involves stabbing joints. Joints are considered primary targets for bayonet thrusting attacks for several reasons:

Cutting the joints immediately incapacitates or cripples the opponent—shocking his system as well.

Joints are connectors (e.g., shoulder to arm, hip to leg) that provide mobility to the limbs. Because they have to be free to do their job, they tend not to be covered by protective gear or clothing.

The range of motion of joints is less than that of the corresponding limbs. Because they are more stationary, they tend to be easier targets.

Recognizing the vulnerability of the joints, xingyi utilizes what is known as *circular wiping motions* for blocking, deflecting, and countering attacks to these areas. In the next technique, the wiping motion is used not only as a block but also as a simultaneous attack to the groin area.

# THRUSTING III

**Action #1** (Figure 3-25): Imagine the opponent thrusts to your chest. Turn your left hand and execute a wiping motion to the front right position. This causes the rifle to thrust diagonally downward. Step forward with the left foot and immediately follow this with the right foot, stepping forward and through.

As your right foot comes to rest in the forward position, flip both hands over and align

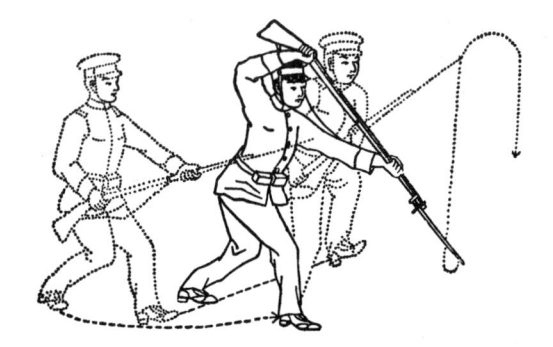

Figure 3-25.

them with your lead foot. Stretch your front hand out in line with the stomach. Bend your right elbow slightly and position it near your forehead. The body of your rifle forms an angle [sloped shape].

**Action #2** (Figure 3-26, *left side of illustration*): Move your rifle from right to left. Lead hand makes a semi-circular movement approximately 180 degrees. The body of the rifle is in a horizontal position and is aligned with lead hand and left knee. As your hand makes its movement, step forward with the left foot. Power and force in both hands should be equal. Eyes are on the opponent.

**Action #3** (Figure 3-26, *right side of illustration*): This movement is similar to the action described earlier *(and shown in Figure 3-19)*. However, when your right foot moves forward, the distance between (*your*) feet should be greater.

**Action #4** (Figure 3-27): This is the same as the action described earlier *(and shown in Figure 3-20)*.

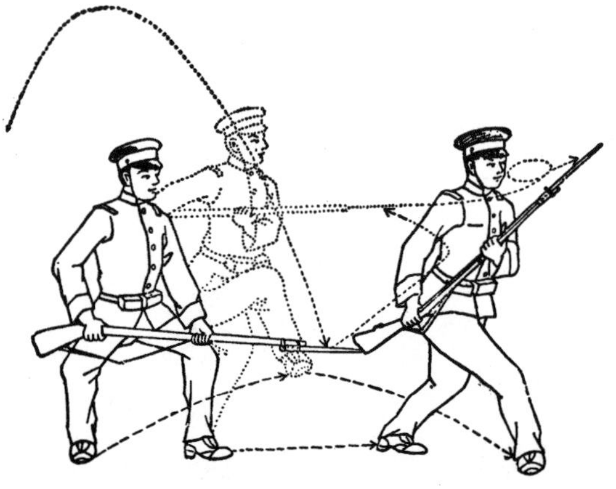

Figure 3-26.

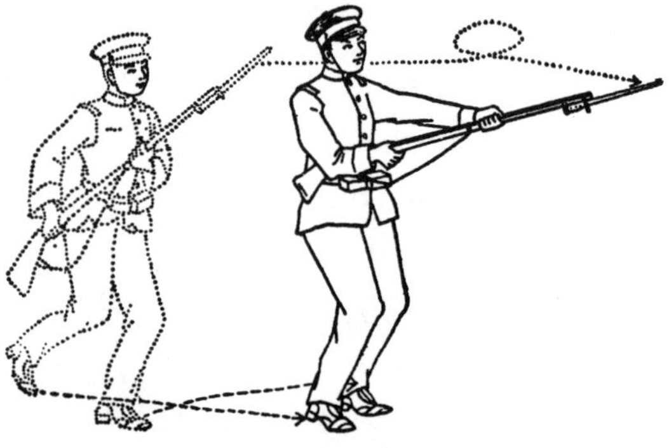

Figure 3-27.

# DRILLS FOR THRUSTING III
## Two-Person Drill (Fixed Position)

Face your opponent while standing at attention.

When the instructor gives the verbal signal "ready," assume a *left forward trinity posture*. Continue to face each other and make sure that you are both slightly out of each other's range.

On a verbal signal from your instructor, your opponent attacks with a straight thrust to your stomach or groin area.

Counter this thrust by executing the wiping motion.

As you block, step with your right foot. Immediately step through and execute a counterattack by using a straight thrust to your opponent's stomach or groin area.

Step back to the starting position and repeat this attack and counterattack sequence for a set number of repetitions.

After one set is completed, reverse roles. You become the attacker while your opponent defends and counters.

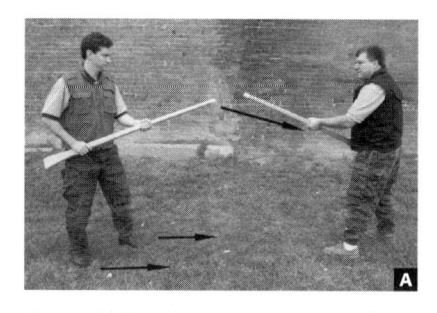

Figure 3-28a. Your opponent attacks with a straight thrust or horizontal slash to your midsection.

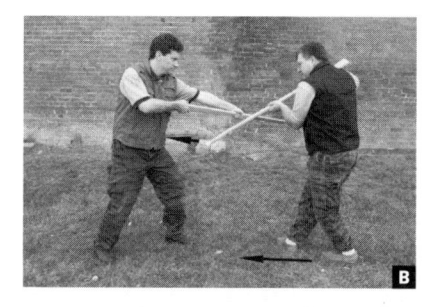

Figure 3-28b. Cross-step and execute a wiping motion. Immediately follow this with a straight thrust to your opponent's midsection or groin.

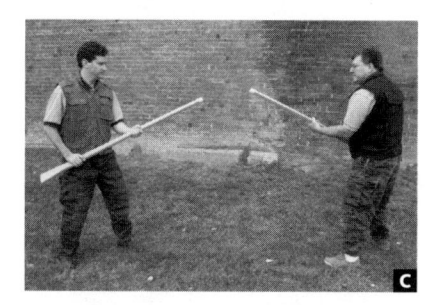

Figure 3-28c. You both step back to the starting position. Repeat the exercise or reverse roles.

## Linear Movement Two-Person Drill

Stand at attention and face your opponent.

When the instructor gives the verbal signal "ready," assume a left forward trinity posture. Continue to face each other and make sure that you are both slightly out of each other's range of attack.

On a verbal signal from your instructor, your partner attacks with a straight thrust to your stomach or groin area.

Counter this thrust by executing the wiping motion.

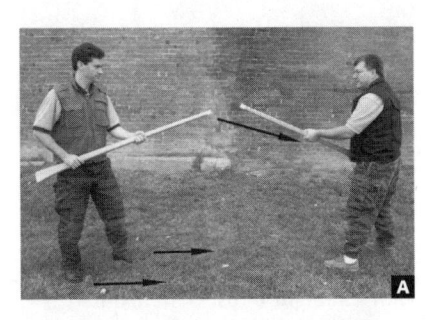

Figure 3-29a. Your opponent attacks with a straight thrust or horizontal slash to your midsection.

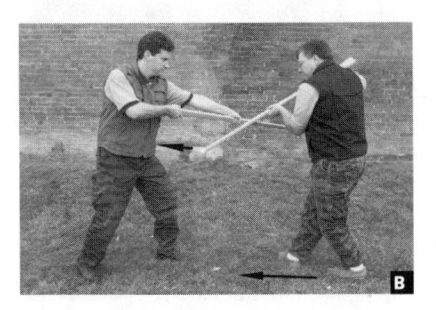

Figure 3-29b. Cross-step and execute a wiping motion. You immediately follow this with a straight thrust to your opponent's midsection or groin.

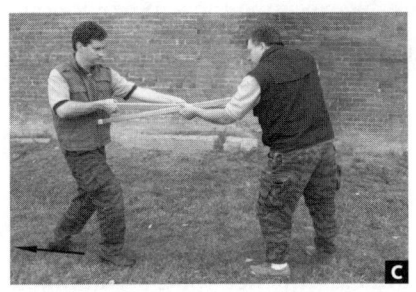

Figure 3-29c. To avoid the thrust, your opponent steps back—first with the lead foot and then with his rear foot. Your opponent then repeats his attack.

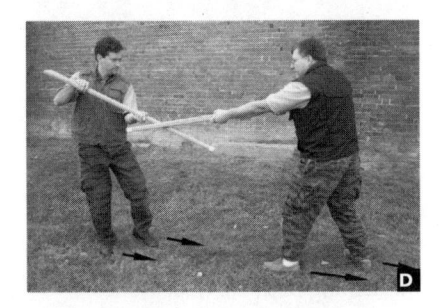

Figure 3-29d. To change direction, your opponent assumes a back stance (after stepping). He blocks your thrust using a wiping motion and steps forward to counterattack.

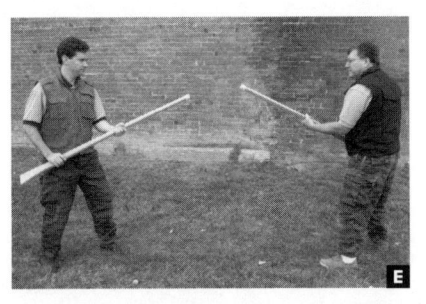

Figure 3-29e. Return to ready position and/or reverse roles.

As you block, step with your right foot. Immediately step through and execute a counterattack by using a straight thrust to your opponent's stomach or groin area.

Your opponent immediately moves back and prepares for another attack. Continue to move forward down the practice area.

Once you have moved the length of the practice area, reverse roles. Continue back and forth along the length of the practice area for an agreed-upon number of repetitions.

## APPLICATIONS OF THRUSTING III

In order to clearly understand the sequence of movements in Figures 3-25 to 3-27 (which shows the finishing thrust), we need to first break down each movement and analyze all of them in terms of specific application. Once this is done we can recombine the movements into the training sequence.

### First Application: Blocking

Your opponent executes a thrust at your waist level or lower.

You block his attack by flipping your rifle and deflecting his weapon to your lower right side.

As you block, step forward with your right foot. Immediately close the distance by stepping forward with your left foot. Thrust into his stomach or groin. (Here we have used real rifles with bayonets to more clearly show the cutting actions.)

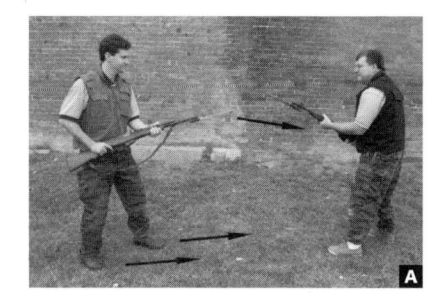

Figure 3-30a. Your opponent attacks with a midsection thrust or slash.

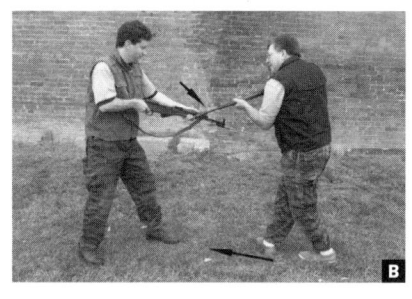

Figure 3-30b. Flip your rifle over and deflect his weapon to your lower right side. Try to cut or smash his lead hand.

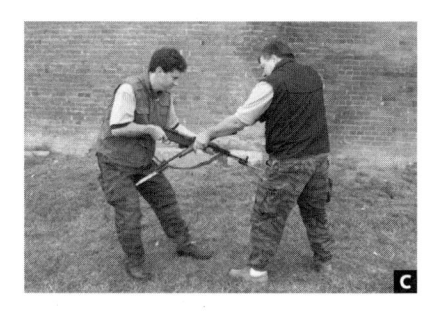

Figure 3-30c. Thrust into his stomach or groin.

## Second Application: Slashing

You have successfully blocked a straight thrust to the right side of your stomach, using a wrist rolling action and body turn to the right.

You counterattack by executing the wiping motion and slashing your opponent on the inside of the thigh of his lead leg.

Alternatively, you execute the wiping motion and thrust into his groin.

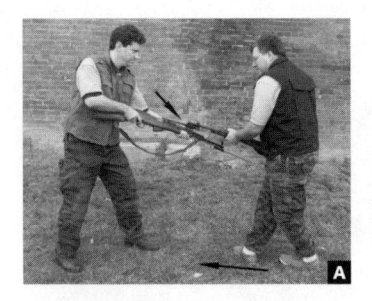

Figure 3-31a. Block the straight thrust or slash to your right side by dropping your blade on your opponent's rifle or lead hand.

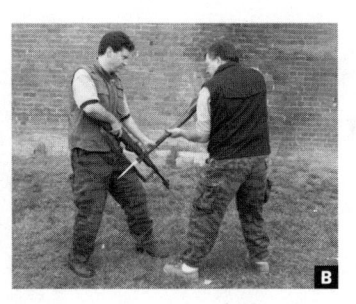

Figure 3-31b. Counterattack with a slash to the inside of his leg.

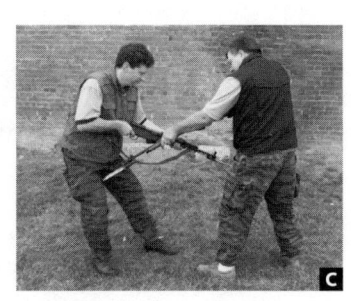

Figure 3-31c. Or thrust into his groin or leg.

## Third Application: Slashing and Thrusting

You successfully blocked a straight thrust to your waist area or lower by using the wiping motion.

To protect himself, your opponent withdraws his attack.

You step through and execute a straight thrust to his stomach or groin.

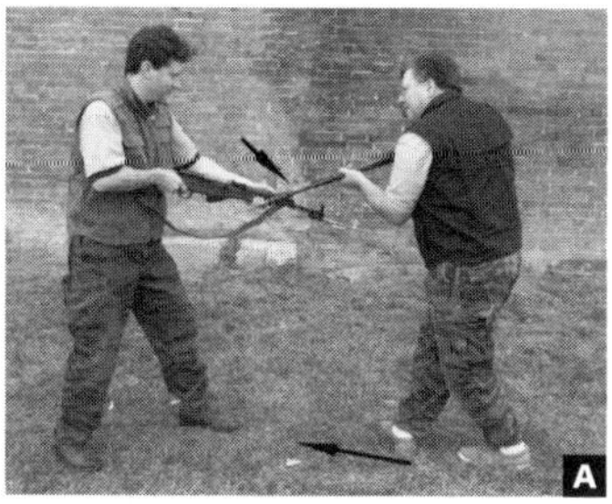

Figure 3-32a. Block a low thrust or slash using a wiping motion.

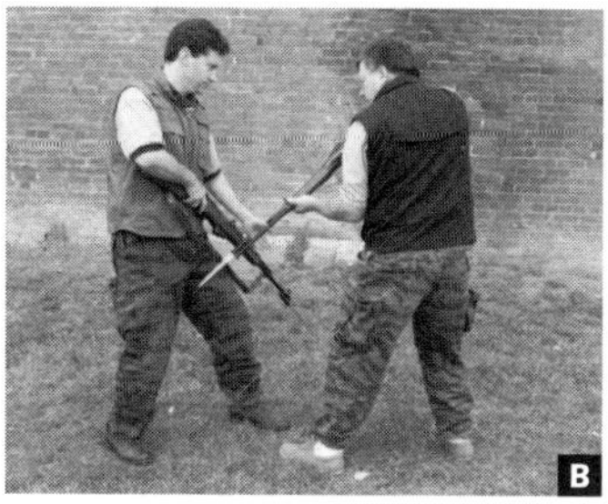

Figure 3-32b. Counter with a slash to the inside of your opponent's leg.

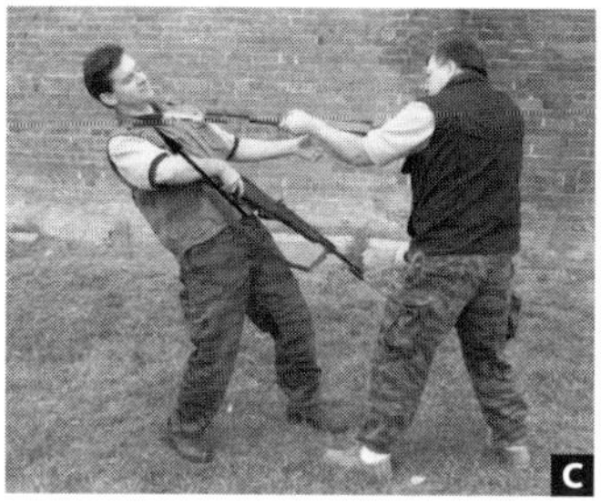

Figure 3-32c. Immediately follow with a thrust to your opponent's upper body.

# THRUSTING IV

**Action #1** (Figure 3-33, *left side of illustration*): Assume your opponent thrusts to the right side of your chest. Vigorously "jump" *(use a quick reinforcing step)* a half-step in the front left direction. Position your body so you face front right.

*"Look angrily at the enemy."*

At the same time your body moves, use the butt of the rifle to push from the lower left direction and deflect the opponent's weapon. Your lead hand brushes to the upper right. Strength and force are used so that the bayonet points upward at your enemy's face. The body of the rifle slopes at a 45-degree angle.

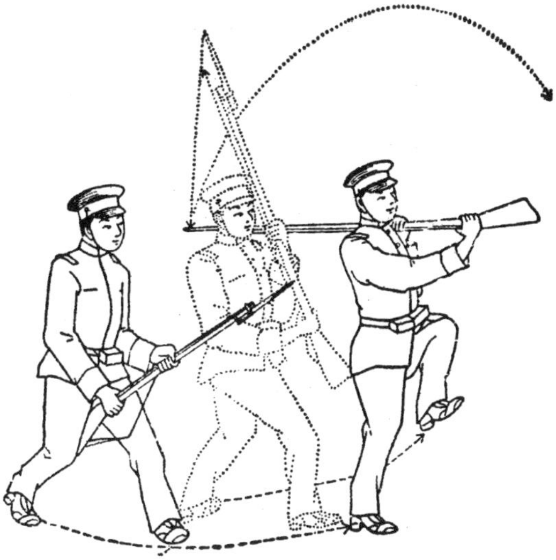

Figure 3-33

## EXPLANATION OF THRUSTING IV
### Ti Guai Li Posture

Western soldiers are taught to use the butts of their rifles to stroke or smash their opponents. This is a totally offensive technique similar to a punch or elbow strike. Xingyi, on the other hand, does not employ this in its repertoire of techniques. Although the so-called *ti guai li* posture superficially resembles a butt stroke, it is neither executed nor employed in the same manner. (This technique, called ti guai li by Huang Po-Nien and others, takes its name from the crippled member of the eight immortals in Chinese mythology. The back-and-forth deflecting action in this maneuver is reminiscent of the motion of the single crutch he used in walking.)

Xingyi-trained soldiers prefer instead to use the cutting edge and point of the bayonet, even in close quarters, as their primary killing weapon. With this strategy in mind, the ti guai li movement becomes a means to an end. Using it, you are able to redirect your opponent's weapon past your body while simultaneously setting him up for a killing blow—all in one continuous movement.

Note: I am not insinuating that the Chinese would never use a butt stroke. In combat you have to exploit every opportunity presented to you. However, one of the primary strategies of xingyi is to always try to move from one position of protection to another position of protection. Understanding this, the idea of lifting your shoulder and exposing your side and armpit in order to strike becomes a less than desirable option.

## APPLICATIONS OF THRUSTING IV

Although the use of the ti guai li movement is not limited by distance (it can be used in extreme close quarters as well as against longer-range attacks), it is usually employed in only two instances:

> Your opponent executes a thrust. The vertical motion of your rifle butt carries the attacker's blade past your body. You immediately follow with a downward slash and thrust.

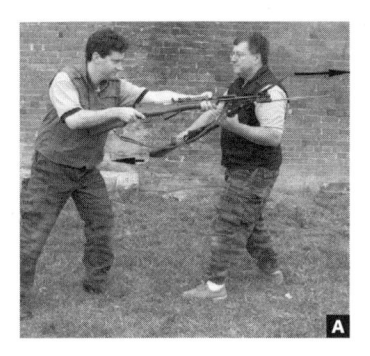

Figure 3-34a. Use a horizontal sweeping action to move the opponent's bayonet past your body.

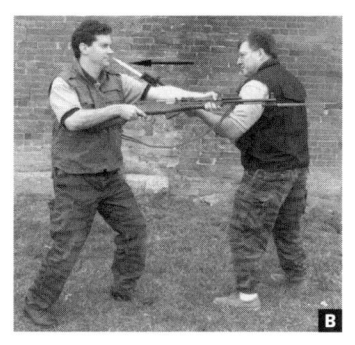

Figure 3-34b. Immediately counter with a slash to his face.

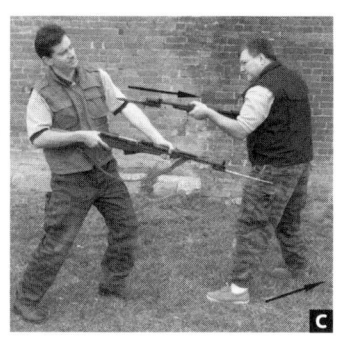

Figure 3-34c. Slice your opponent's lead arm or hand as you withdraw your blade.

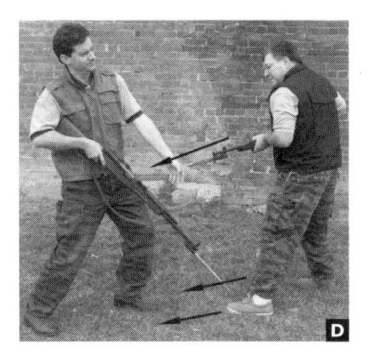

Figure 3-34d. Chop down on his lead arm and position your body for the thrust.

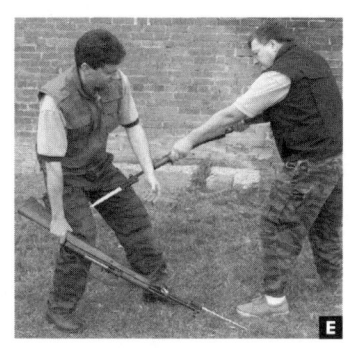

Figure 3-34e. Thrust to his groin or inside of the leg.

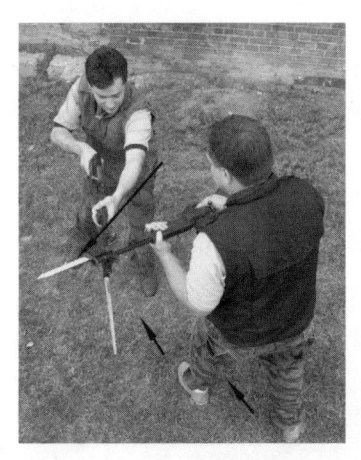

Figure 3-35. Over-the-shoulder view of the horizontal redirection action. (Remember to close distance as you block.)

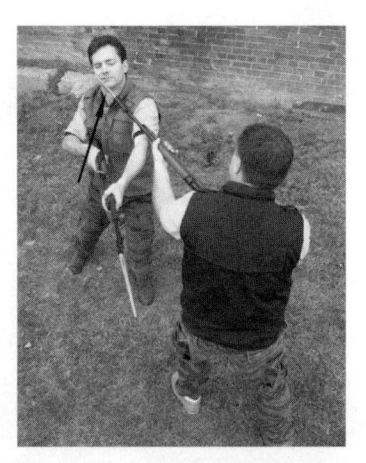

Figure 3-36. Horizontal slash or thrust to your opponent's neck or face. (The distance between attacker and defender in this photograph is exaggerated for clarity.)

Your opponent rushes you. Again, the vertical motion moves his weapon past you. You immediately follow up with a strike, using the butt of your rifle coupled with a hip-waist turn. Next, you deliver the finishing moves—a slash and thrust, in quick succession.

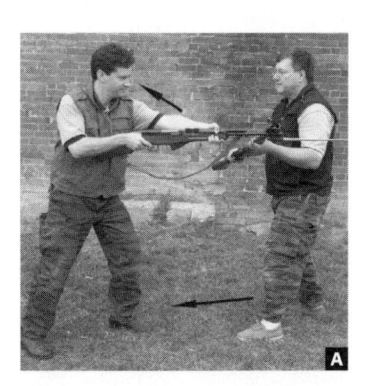

Figure 3-37a. As your opponent charges, redirect his weapon past your body and close the distance.

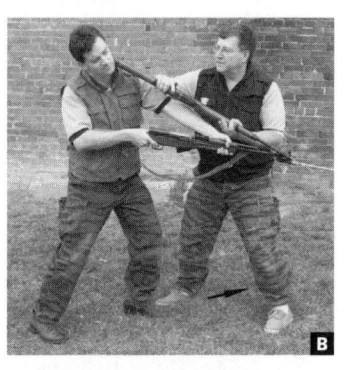

Figure 3-37b. As you step in, strike with the butt of your weapon. (Stepping and striking are done in one continuous movement.)

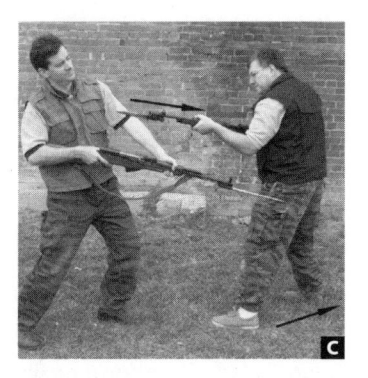

Figure 3-37c. Slash his arm as you withdraw your blade.

Chapter Three **91**

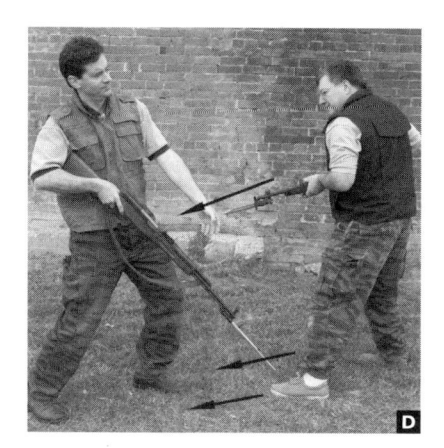

Figure 3-37d. Redirect your attack to his midsection.

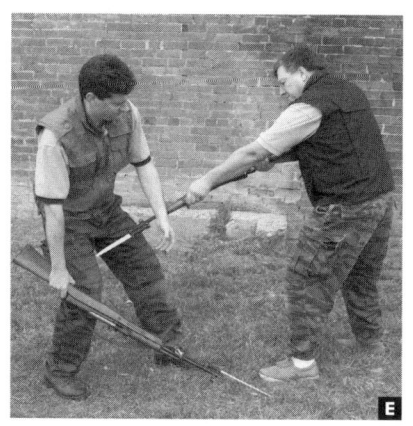

Figure 3-37e. Stab him in the stomach, leg, or groin.

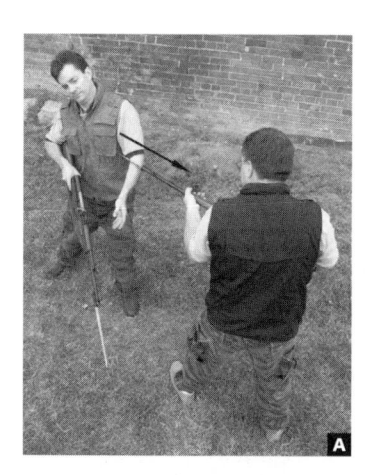

Figure 3-38a. Over-the-shoulder shot showing the arm slash.

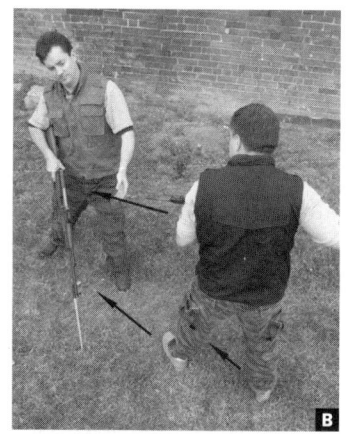

Figure 3-38b. Note the angle at which the counterattack is delivered.

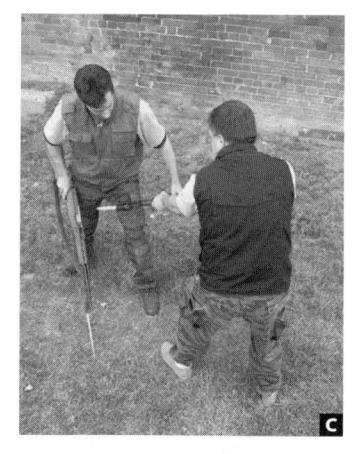

Figure 3-38c. The groin and legs have little or no protection, making them vulnerable to attack.

## THRUSTING IV (CONTINUED)

**Action #2** (Figure 3-33, *right side of illustration*): With right foot forward, first vigorously lift your left foot. Use whichever hand is at the back to push the butt of the rifle to the front *(forward and away from the body)*. Trigger guard now faces up. Bayonet points to the back. Elbows are tight against the sides of the body. This is known as ti guai li position.

**Action #3** (Figure 3-39, *left side of illustration*): Take a large step forward with the left foot, *(a distance)* approximately 3 feet in length. Arms hang down with elbows almost straight. As both feet come to rest (approximately 2 feet apart), chop at the enemy. The rifle should face the right.

**Action #4** (Figure 3-39, *right side of illustration*): Move the left foot slightly back. Stamp the right foot. This helps to accelerate the stepping action of the left foot. As you step, turn both hands over. Raise the lead arm to shoulder height. Position your back hand above the head. Thrust with force to the upper part of the enemy's body. This posture is known as *smooth style pounding rifle*.

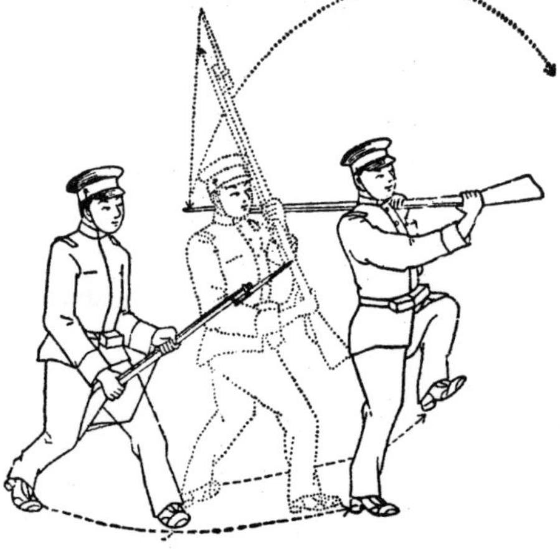

Figure 3-33

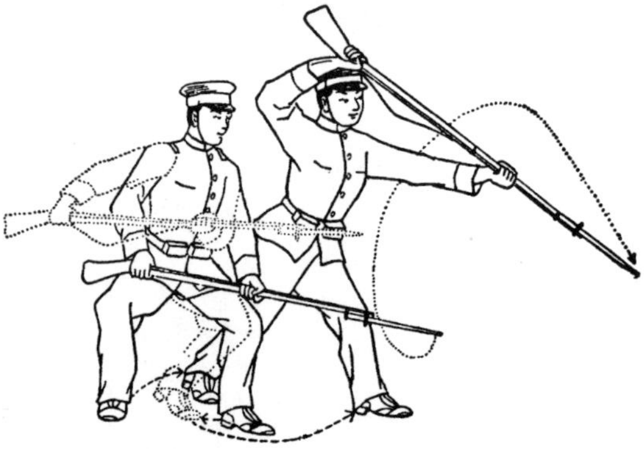

Figure 3-39

Chapter Three

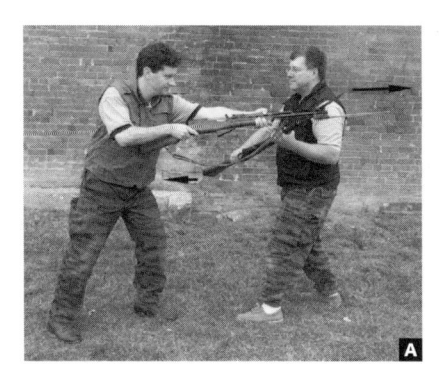

Figure 3-40a. Use ti guai li to redirect your opponent's weapon past your body.

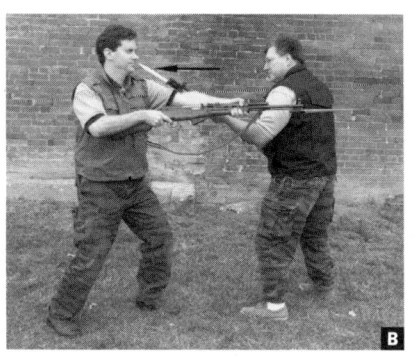

Figure 3-40b. Slash his face or throat.

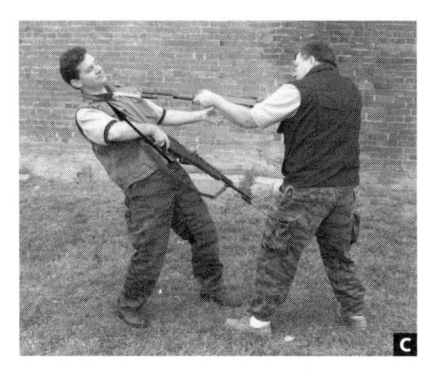

Figure 3-40c. Or thrust into his throat or upper body.

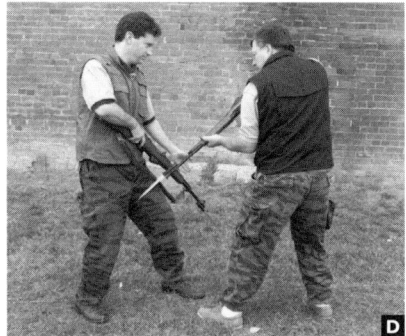

Figure 3-40d. Follow with a wiping motion or slash to his leg or groin.

# TEN CONTINUOUS FLOWING ACTIONS

**Action #1** (Figure 3-41): Imagine that your opponent thrusts at your chest. Make a circular movement with your left hand, downward from left to right. Step forward with the left foot and thrust vigorously to the front with your right hand. Right foot stamps the ground *(steps firmly and stabilizes the weight)* and lands parallel to the ankle of the front foot. Hold your rifle in line with, and tightly to, the chest. Bayonet faces right. This action forms a *crushing style stance*.

**Action #2** (Figure 3-42): Assume your opponent is thrusting at your left arm. Use your left hand to make a circular deflecting motion with the rifle. Immediately thrust from the upper left direction to front right position. As you execute the thrust, quickly step backward with your right foot. Your left foot follows and is placed behind the right leg. This action is either called *stepping backward stance* or *scissor hip* (cross) *stance*. Left hand holds the rifle at an angle with the point of the bayonet approximately 10 inches from the ground. Right hand tightly touches the right hip bone. This posture is known as *back step chop rifle*.

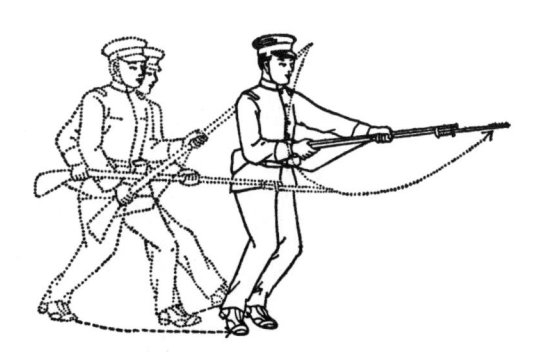

Figure 3-41.

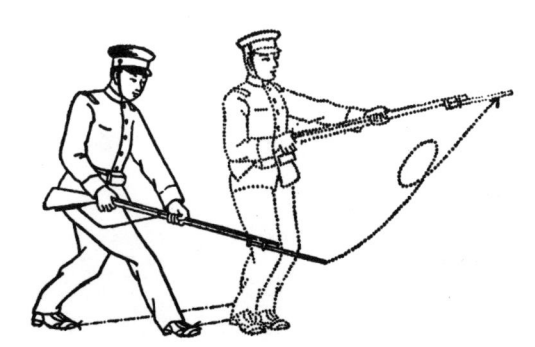

Figure 3-42.

**Action #3** (Figure 3-43): Vigorously step forward with your right foot. Your left foot stamps and lands approximately 1 foot behind the front foot. As you step, use your left palm to hold the butt of the rifle against your abdomen. Use force to point the bayonet to the right. Thrust at your opponent's heart. This action is called *smooth style crushing rifle*.

**Action #4** (Figure 3-44, *left side of illustration*): Assume the opponent thrusts to your right side *(midsection or stomach height)*. Quickly step backward with the left foot, and pivot it slightly. Right foot follows with another step backward. As you step, use both hands to quickly snap the rifle downward. Bayonet and stomach align. This action will cause the opponent's weapon to be positioned beneath your rifle. Immediately follow this technique with Action #5.

**Action #5** (Figure 3-44, *right side of illustration*): Action #5 is similar to Action #3. The difference here is that the stepping and thrusting actions are done at the same time. Also, both hands are together to hold and lift the rifle.

Your left foot takes a large and vigorous step so the tip of the bayonet automatically points to the enemy's stomach. This maneuver is called *step thrust*. Although very practical, you need strong wrists to effectively execute this technique.

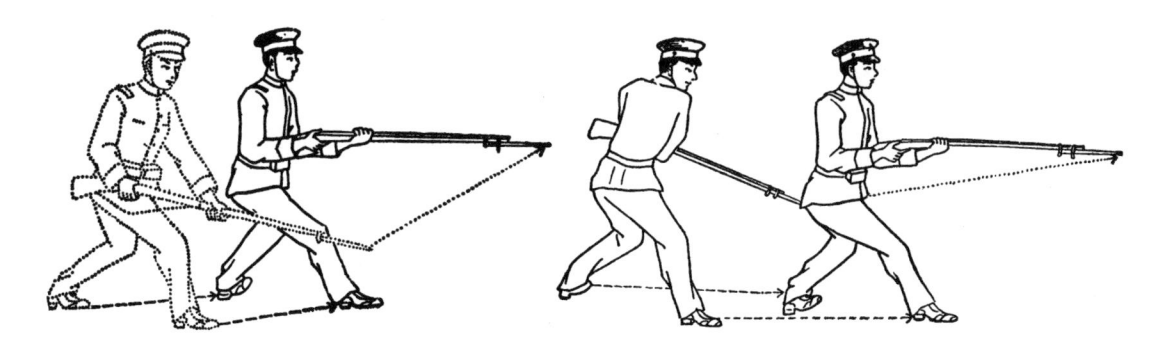

Figure 3-43.

Figure 3-44.

**Action #6** (Figure 3-45): Assume your opponent is thrusting to your chest. Use your left hand to point the tip of the rifle downward at an angle. Quickly snap *(or wipe)* to the front right direction. As you snap, step forward with the left foot. Follow by stepping with the right foot, placing it ahead of the left. Your left wrist is palm up. Turn or flip the rifle, putting hands, eyes, and foot in one line. *(Your left hand is level with the stomach.)* Next, turn the wrist of your right hand to the outside and raise it to your right temple. When completed, the bayonet should point at an angle toward the enemy. *(The bayonet should be angled approximately 45°. The target areas are either the inside of the upper legs or the groin.)* This is called *pounding rifle stance*.

**Action #7** (Figure 3-46): Action #7 is almost the same as Action #2 (Figure 3-42), except that the left foot steps backward to land in front of the right foot. This becomes a *chop rifle step*. The stance forms a *ba* [Chinese numeral 8] shape, with your feet approximately 1½ feet apart. This is called a *backward step horizontal rifle*.

**Action #8** (Figure 3-47): Assume your opponent thrusts at your left shoulder joint. Utilizing both hands, simultaneously raise your front hand while dropping your back hand. Couple this action with a horizontal snap to the left and a forceful, powerful upward drilling action.

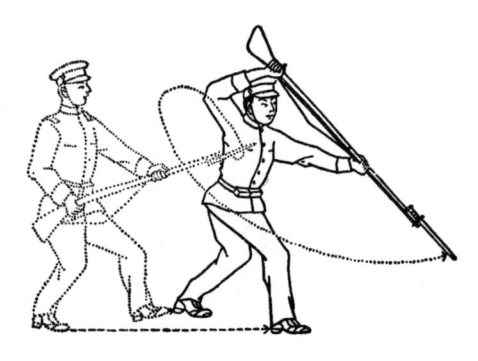

Figure 3-45.

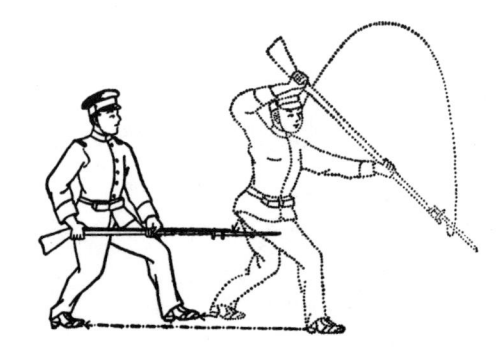

Figure 3-46.

Quickly step forward with your left foot and follow with your right. The body of the rifle and your left elbow are held tightly together.

Pivot the bayonet at an angle toward the enemy. This deflects his weapon to the left. This is called *drilling rifle method*.

**Action #9** (Figure 3-48): Your opponent thrusts at your abdomen. Use both hands to hold your rifle and point it downward. Lift your left foot. Take a big step forward with your right foot and redirect the opponent's weapon to the right. While your opponent is unprepared, plant the left foot and thrust at his abdomen. This technique is called *slash toward the coming wind*.

**Action #10** (Figure 3-49): Action #10 is the same as Action #1 (Figure 3-41).

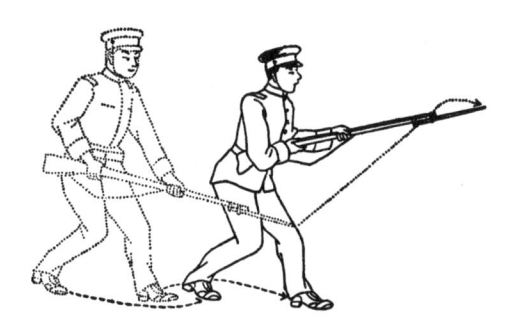

Figure 3-47.

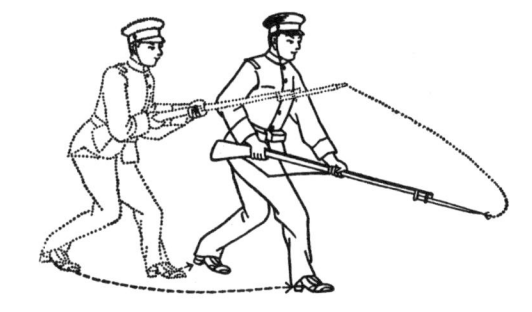

Figure 3-48.

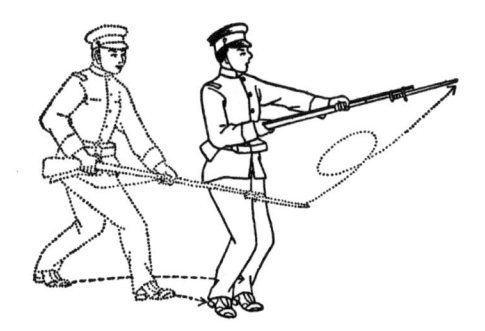

Figure 3-49.

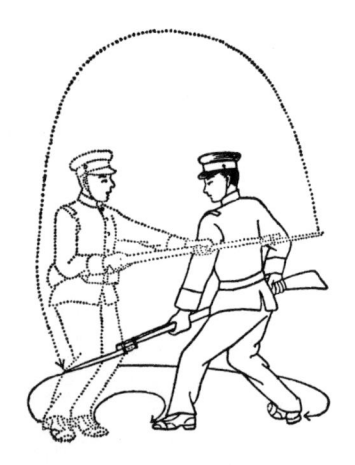

# TURNING AROUND

**Action #11** (Figure 3-50): Assume the opponent attacks from the rear. Use a small and unobtrusive step to move your left foot in the front right direction. Hold the rifle up with both hands. Make a right turn to the back. Turn your rifle 180 degrees and immediately chop the opponent's lead hand. This movement is called *detach* (or escape) *changing* (or exchanging) *shadows*.

Figure 3-50.

# EXPLANATION OF TEN CONTINUOUS FLOWING ACTIONS

The ten continuous flowing actions as described by Huang are essentially the five element linking form for rifle and bayonet. Because Huang's writings contain both a description of each movement and an application, there is some confusion in understanding the text. To make the sequence easier to learn, I have added, in this section, a simplified description of the flowing actions (complete with photographs). They are numbered here, to indicate a sequence of flow of the actions.

1. Stand at attention (Figure 3-51).
2. Assume ready position (Figure 3-52).
3. Make a circular movement downward from left to right (Figure 3-53).
4. Step forward with your left foot and thrust straight ahead (Figure 3-54). Although this is a high thrust, the elbows are kept low and close to your body.

Chapter Three 99

5. Make a circular movement to the left to block a thrust to your left arm (Figure 3-55).
6. Make a horizontal slash from left to right (Figure 3-56).
7. Step backward with your right foot and follow with your left foot (cross stance). The knees should not be locked. The space between the knees should be approximately the width of your fist (Figures 3-57a and 3-57b).
8. Immediately drop the point of your rifle toward the ground (Figure 3-58). Slash to the inside of your opponent's lead leg.

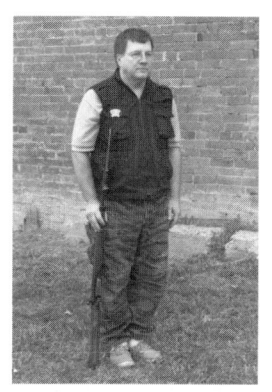

Figure 3-51.

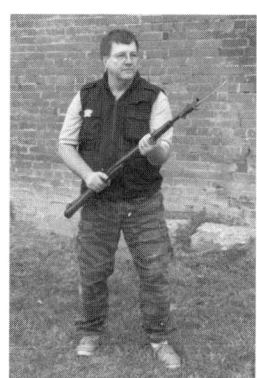

Figure 3-52.

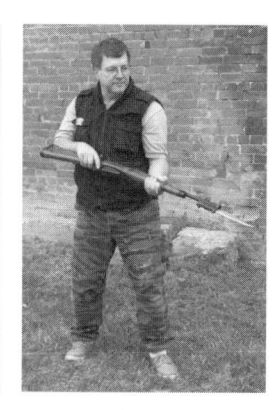

Figure 3-53.

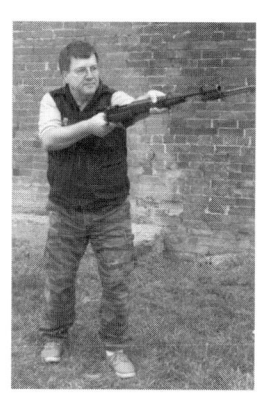

Figure 3-54.

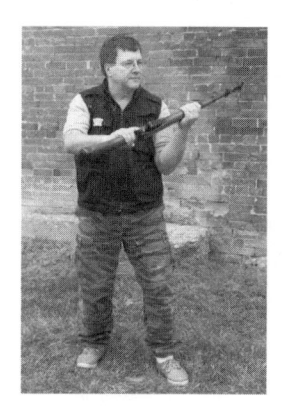

Figure 3-55.

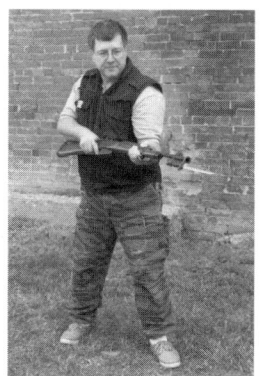

Figure 3-56.

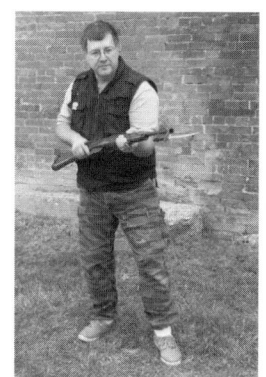

Figure 3-57a.

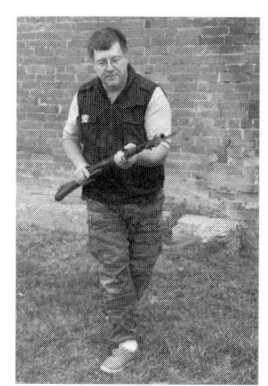

Figure 3-58b.

9. Step forward with your right foot and reinforce this step with your left foot. Thrust your bayonet at your opponent's heart (Figure 3-59).
10. Step backward with your left foot. Quickly follow with your right foot (Figure 3-60).
11. Snap the rifle downward (Figure 3-60). Imagine catching your opponent's rifle below yours.
12. Use a circular arm motion to turn your body and your rifle to the left (Figure 3-61).
13. Step-thrust (Figure 3-62). Shuffle-step with right foot forward to opponent's stomach.
14. Step forward into ready position (Figure 3-63).
15. Execute a wiping motion to the front right direction. As you wipe, step forward with your left foot. Follow this with a quick diagonal step to the right, as in pounding fist (Figure 3-64).
16. Step backward with your right foot and draw your left foot in front of the right foot. As you step, flip your rifle back to a horizontal position. Face it toward the front (Figure 3-65).
17. Execute a straight thrust (Figure 3-66). (In this illustration the lead arm has been raised to show how to rotate for the thrusting action.) The lead hand ends up on top.
18. Perform a basic blocking action (Figure 3-67).
19. Execute a straight thrust with the left-foot reinforcing step (Figure 3-68).
20. Take a short step with your left foot. Step through with your right foot and block down on your opponent's lead hand (Figure 3-69).
21. Thrust at your opponent's groin (Figure 3-70).

Chapter Three 101

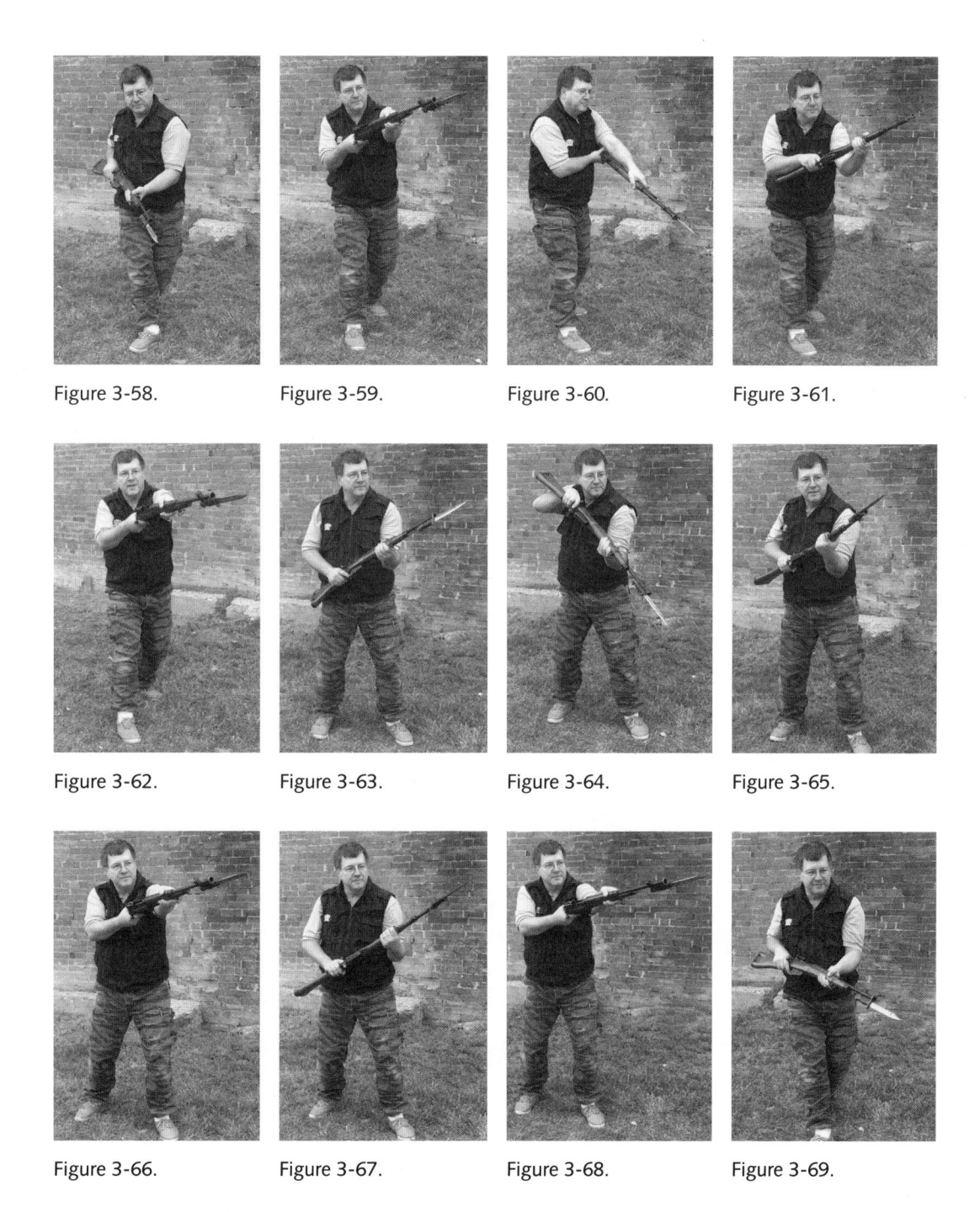

Figure 3-58.

Figure 3-59.

Figure 3-60.

Figure 3-61.

Figure 3-62.

Figure 3-63.

Figure 3-64.

Figure 3-65.

Figure 3-66.

Figure 3-67.

Figure 3-68.

Figure 3-69.

22. Use your rifle to make a circular movement from the lower left to upper right position (Figure 3-71).
23. Bring your feet together and thrust (Figures 3-72a and 3-72b).
24. Take a small step with your left foot and move it to the front right direction. Make a right turn and land with your left foot in front (Figure 3-73).
25. Chop down with your rifle (Figure 3-74).
26. Finish, or repeat the form in the opposite direction.

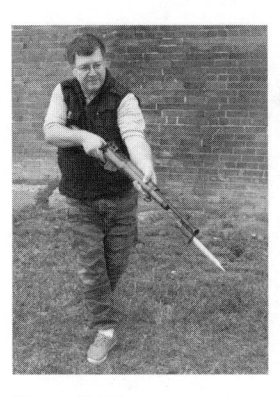

Figure 3-70.

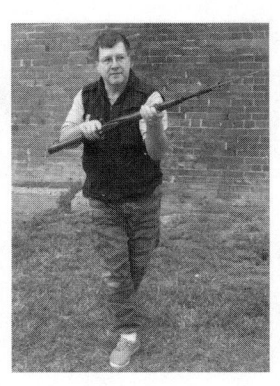

Figure 3-71.

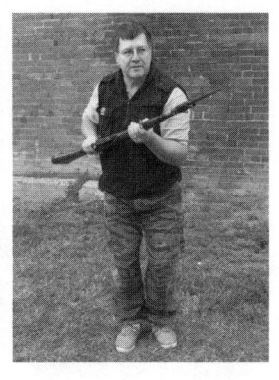

Figure 3-72a.

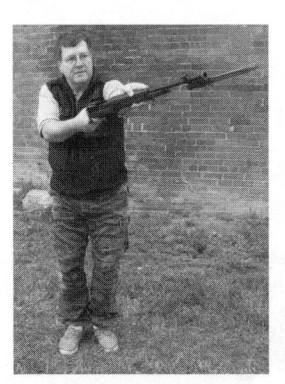

Figure 3-72b.

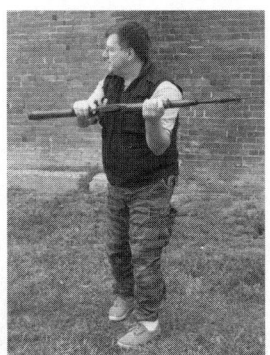

Figure 3-73.

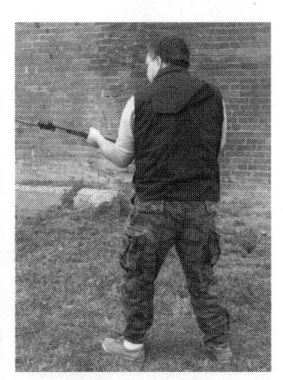

Figure 3-74.

# Chapter 4

## COMMON MISCONCEPTIONS REGARDING THE XINGYI MILITARY SABRE

As we look at the original diagrams and photos in this chapter, we see the weapon being used is a Western-style army officer's sabre. This was the standard solo practice weapon for military xingyi.

## No Dadao

Recently, reference has been made in articles and on the Internet to the xingyi *dadao* (big knife) method. This weapon was made famous by the 29th army corps and other units during the war with Japan. One author (who shall remain nameless) states that the use of the dadao in military xingyi precedes the straight sabre. He also states (and I'm paraphrasing here) that the straight sabre only came into use because of the unavailability of the dadao for training. These statements have no basis in fact. Having looked at a broad cross-section of xingyi writings and illustrated manuals published during the early part of the twentieth century, I found:

- No illustrations of xingyi sabre methods using the dadao
- No mention of the dadao in xingyi training (historically or otherwise)
- That Huang and others discuss the use of the *upper hanging method* while on horseback. Since the dadao is strictly an infantry weapon, it would have no practical use in the cavalry.

No evidence that the dadao was taught at the Central Military Academy. As well, since this academy and others were modeled on Western military academies, the common cutting weapon those officers would carry is the straight military sabre.

Moreover, when I questioned the author of the previously mentioned article, he was unable to offer any evidence to support his statements.

This is not to say that xingyi techniques were not used in the dadao units. Given the ease of adapting such methods, it is almost a certainty. However, the evidence points to the straight sabre methods having been used first and those for the dadao second, and not the other way around.

## No Miaodao

Another type of sabre erroneously associated with the Central Military Academy at Nanjing is the *miaodao* (corn leaf or sprout sabre). Some contemporary instructors even claim to teach the Central Military Academy's miaodao form. This claim is completely false. Not only was the miaodao *not* taught at the academy, it was also never part of the standard curriculum at the Nanjing Zhong Yang Guoshu Guan (Nanjing Central/National Martial Arts Academy).

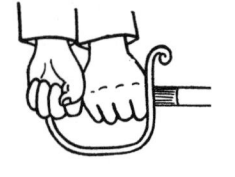

Figure 4-1. Holding sabre pose.

## Final Comment

Included as part of Col. Chang's teaching curriculum was a xingyi-based straight sword form adaptable for use with the straight sabre. Although I have practiced it for more than thirty-five years, I have not heard it discussed outside of its military context. It differs significantly from and should not be confused with the *san cai jian* (three talents sword) method taught by Xu Shi-Jin at the Wuhan branch of the Central Military Academy.

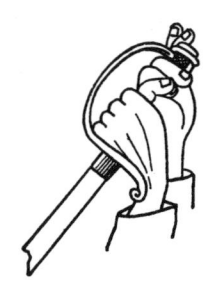

Figure 4-2. Raising sabre pose.

Chapter Four

# IMPORTANT FUNDAMENTALS FOR HANDLING THE TWO-HANDED SABRE

Sabre forms are patterned after the five element fists, namely: splitting, crushing, drilling, pounding, and crossing fists. To make the sabre forms simple to learn and practical to use, all of the techniques are based upon the key principles of intercepting, deflecting, cutting the opponent's hand or wrist, chopping, thrusting, hitting, or slicing upward from under the opponent's guard.

Effectiveness of techniques lies in coupling their basic nature with application of both hidden wrist and hidden sabre forms. Although not flowery, these techniques prevent the opponent from utilizing his skill.

## SECTION I: HOLDING SABRE METHOD (FORM)

To make the transition from ready or standing position (Figures 4-3 and 4-3m) to open position, perform the following actions.

Grip the sabre with both hands. Right hand tightly grasps the top part of the handle. Left hand lightly holds the bottom. Sink your Qi. Drop both arms and let your hands touch the lower right side of your stomach. The sabre's blade should point upward at an angle greater

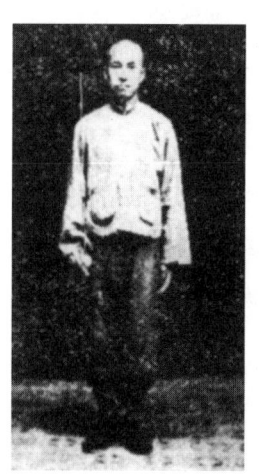

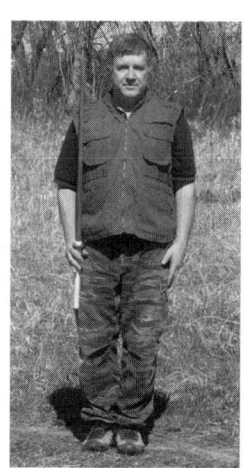

Figure 4-3.   Figure 4-3m.

than 45 degrees. Eyes focus on the tip of the blade. Left foot is forward. Right foot is behind. Right foot gives support by pushing against the floor. This position is the same as splitting fist and is known as *hidden sword position* (Figures 4-4 and 4-4m).

*(In the military method of training you normally step forward with the left foot. Again, the idea here is to teach the soldier to advance rather than retreat. Stepping back with the right foot, however, is equally correct.)*

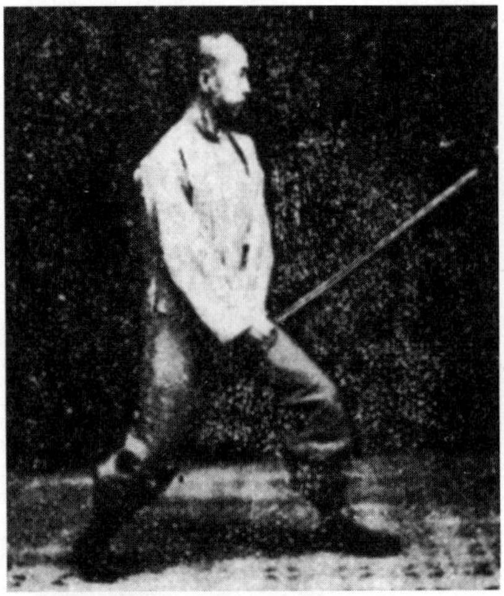

Figure 4-4.

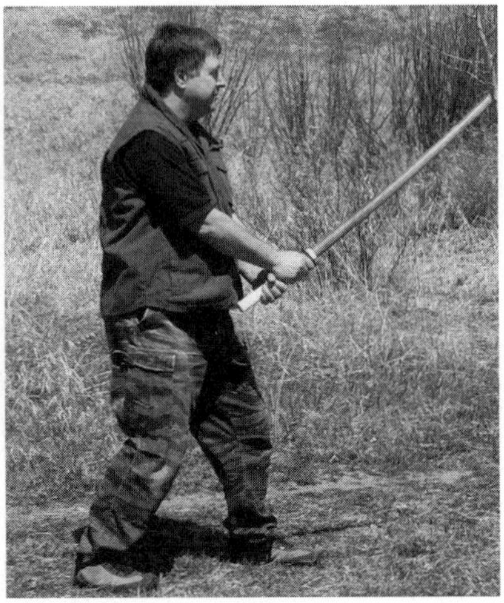

Figure 4-4m.

## SECTION II: CHOPPING SABRE METHOD

To make the transition from open position to *chopping sabre position*, follow the orders:

*"Ready . . . chopping sabre . . . forward . . . go."*

**Action #1** (Figures 4-5, 4-5m1 to 4-5m5 inclusive): Left Position. When you hear the word "go," raise the sabre's handle to your upper left side. Blade is outside of the body *(pointing away from you)*. From this upper left position, slice downward with a direct diagonal strike to your opponent's left side. This technique is called *parting the horse's mane*. It is most suitable for use on horseback.

As you chop, take a slight step forward with your left foot. Step through with the right foot and place it in front. Your right foot should travel approximately 3 feet. Final distance between the two feet should be approximately 20 inches.

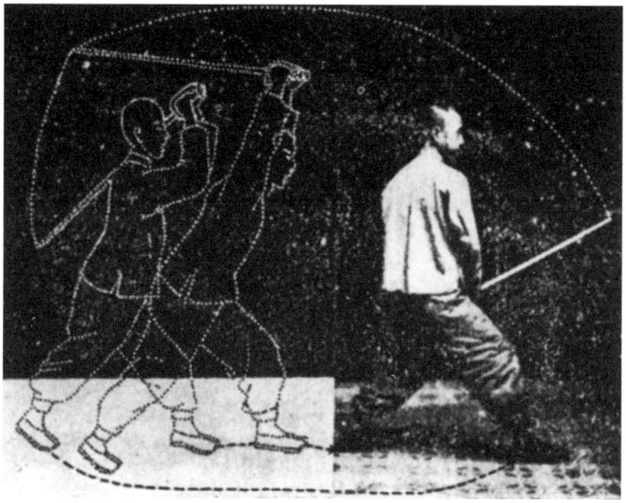

Figure 4-5.

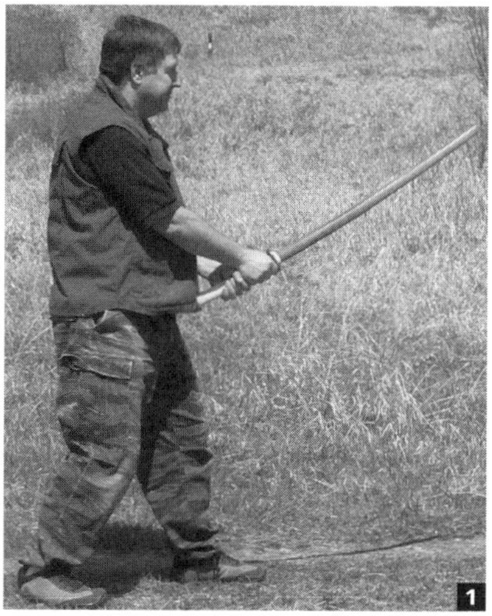

Figure 4-5m1.

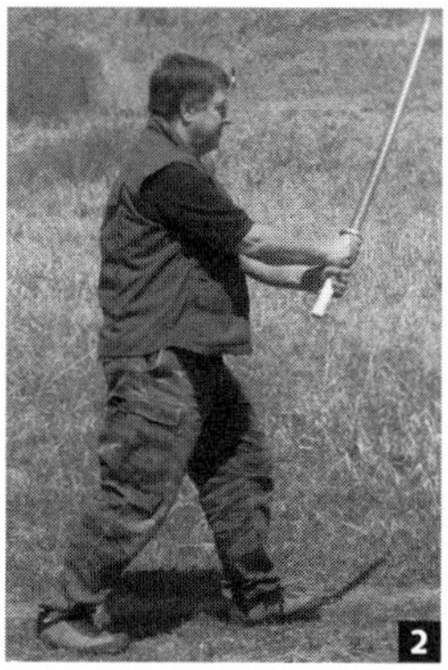

Figure 4-5m2.

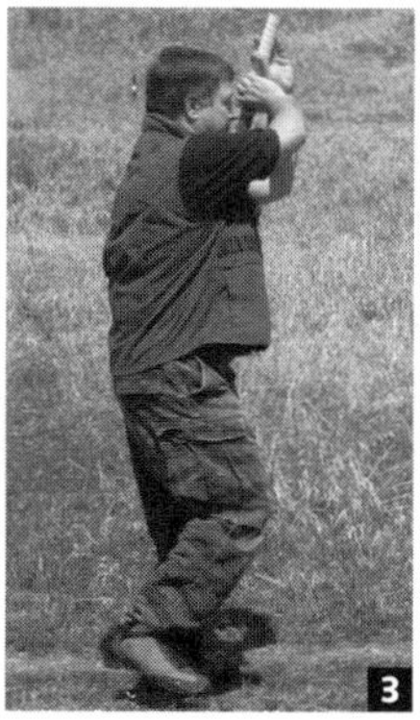

Figure 4-5m3.

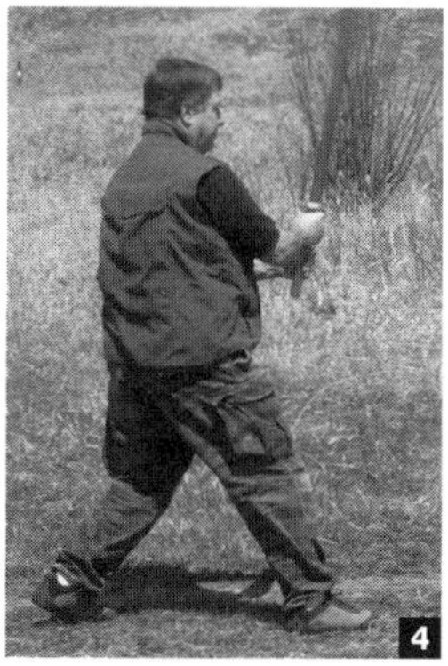

Figure 4-5m4.

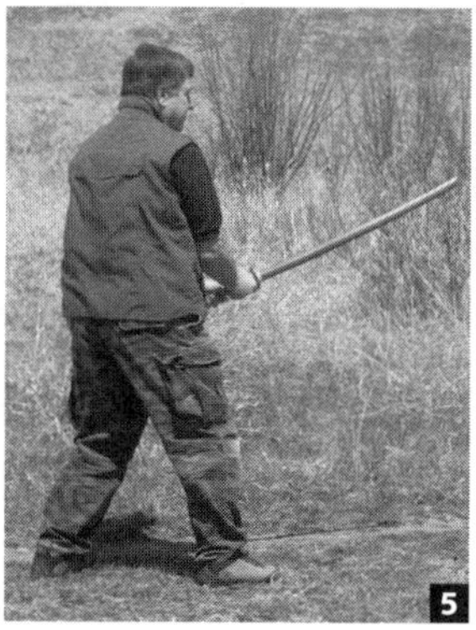

Figure 4-5m5.

## EXPLANATION OF RAISING SABRE POSE

*Raising sabre pose* is a deflection or redirection of a direct attack to either side of your upper body. Typically, this defense is used when your opponent begins the attack outside of your range. For example, your opponent thrusts the bayonet at your left shoulder while charging you.

As we saw in Chapter 3, a properly trained combatant will break the timing between stepping and thrusting. This means you must avoid the tendency to anticipate or react prematurely. It also means you must be able to quickly move your sabre into the blocking position.

### Maximizing Efficiency and Speed

The ability to react quickly is initiated by the hands and not by simply trying to lift the arms. Although Huang uses the phrase "raise the sabre's handle" he is *not* telling us to lift the sabre. Because such an action requires you to lift your arms, it tends to be slow.

Besides being mechanically inefficient, lifting the arms creates three additional problems:

- Lifting the arms commits you to the defense. If the attacker fakes or delays the thrust, or you panic and react too early, you will have placed yourself in a vulnerable position.
- Lifting the arms exposes your body, especially your armpits and side, to attack (Figure 4-6).
- Raising your arms tends to obstruct your vision (Figure 4-7a and 4-7b). This is particularly dangerous if the opponent counters and launches a second attack to your lower body.

### Quick Movement

The key to quick movement is to use your right hand as a fulcrum around which the sabre rotates. Force to move the blade is generated by the pushing action of the left hand, similar to the punch in crush-

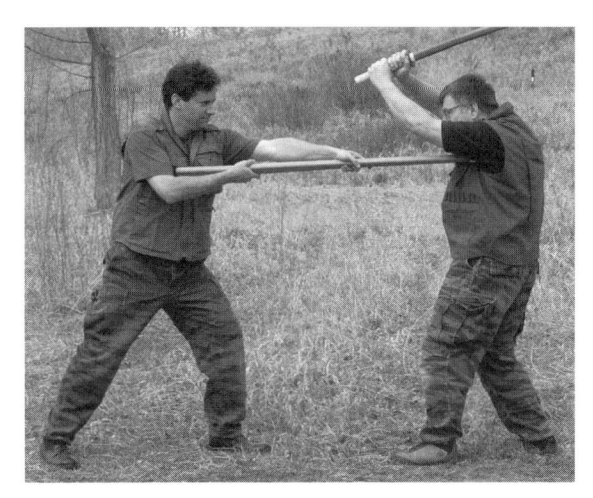

Figure 4-6. Raising your arms exposes your body to attack.

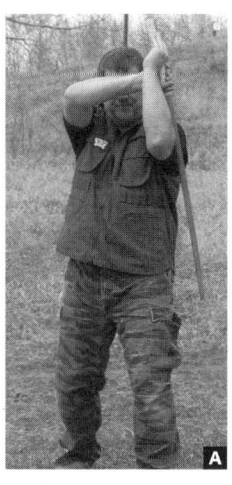

Figure 4-7a. Raising the arm obstructs your vision.

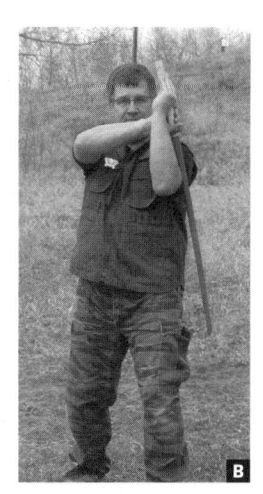

Figure 4-7b. Proper arm position.

ing fist. This movement of the left hand causes the blocking action to commence before you move your arms. The action of the arms is secondary and follows the movement of the hands and blade (Figures 4-8a, 4-8b, and 4-8c).

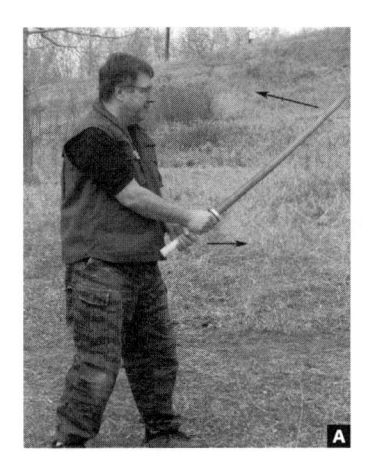

Figure 4-8a. Push out and up with your left hand.

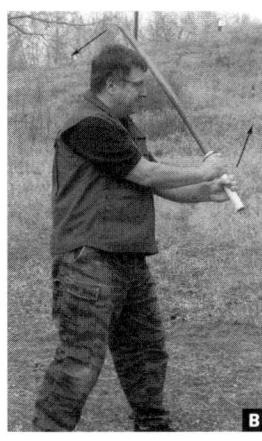

Figure 4-8b. Your right hand acts as a fulcrum.

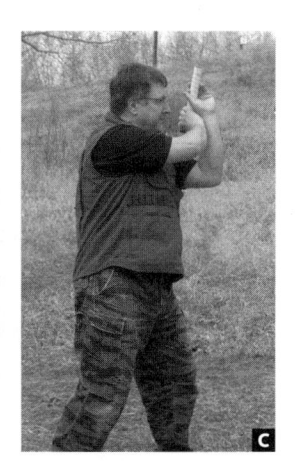

Figure 4-8c. Raised sabre, ready to block or strike.

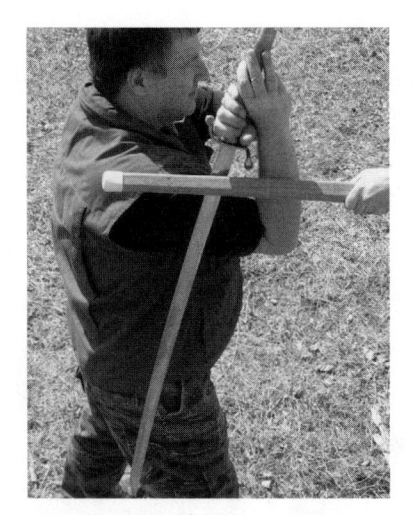

Figure 4-8d. The proper angle of the blade prevents damaging the sabre as you block.

As you can see from this explanation, raising sabre pose is not an attempt to block or knock the attacker's weapon out of the way. Such an action would most likely damage or break your blade. Rather, you are using the side of the blade to guide the opponent's weapon past your body (Figure 4-8d). At the same time you redirect, you also position yourself for the counterattack. It is important to understand that the faster and more committed the opponent's attack is, the easier it is to deflect, making it harder for him to recover.

## APPLICATION OF CHOPPING SABRE METHOD

There are two ways to counterattack using the chopping sabre method. Both begin with the same blocking action. The difference in your strike is related to the relative distance between you and your opponent.

### Counterattack #1

Here are the steps.

**1.** You are standing with your left foot forward (Figure 4-9a).

**2.** Your opponent initiates a bayonet thrust or sword cut to your left shoulder. He is just within range.

**3.** As he thrusts or slashes, execute the raising sabre pose to move his weapon past your body (Figure 4-9b).

**4.** Immediately step straight forward with your right foot and slash diagonally downward (Figure 4-9c). Target areas are the forearms, causing him to drop his weapon, or the exposed side of his neck.

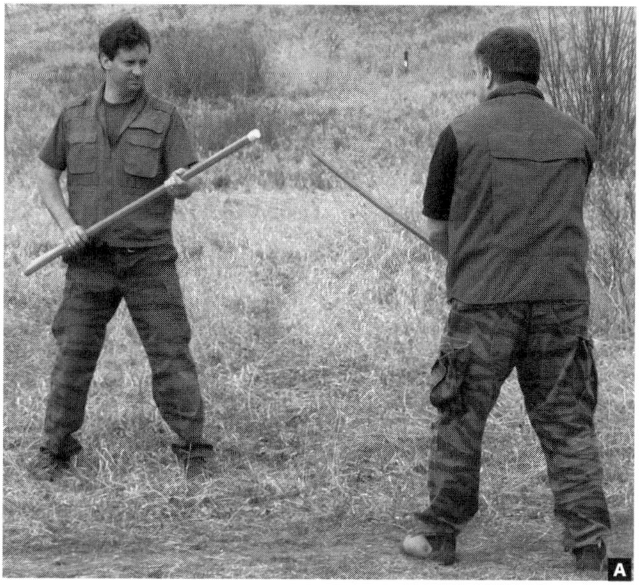

Chapter Four **111**

Figure 4-9a. Opponent is just within range as he thrusts.

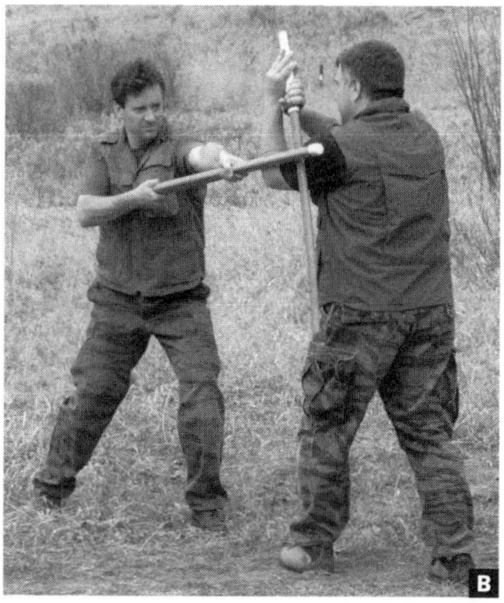

Figure 4-9b. Redirect his attack with a raising sabre pose.

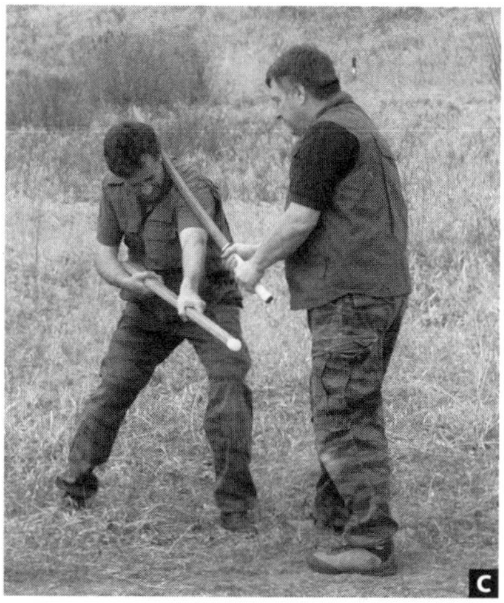

Figure 4-9c. Chop his neck or forearms.

## Straight Step Only

There is a tendency when attacking to step in at an angle and twist or rotate your upper body toward the target as you chop. There are two reasons why this should not be done:

> Twisting prevents much of the force you generate when stepping from being transferred into the target. That is, the turning action causes your arms and sabre to make an arc, which diminishes the momentum of the body and, by extension, the force of the cut (Figure 4-10a).

> Turning your body gives your opponent the opportunity to move and block. As well, his actions are more likely to throw you off balance (Figure 4-10b).

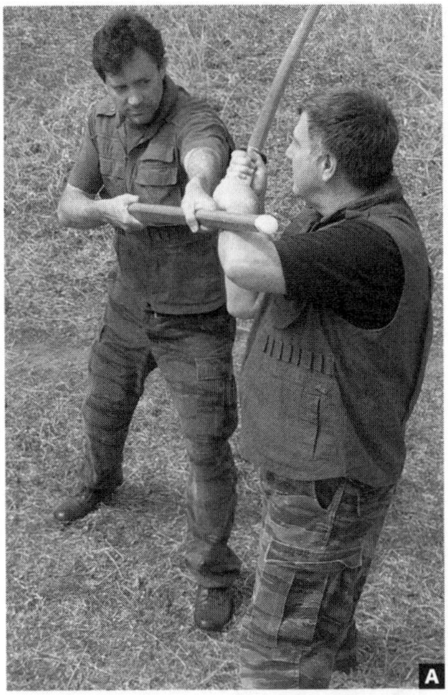

Figure 4-10a. Twisting your body throws you off balance.

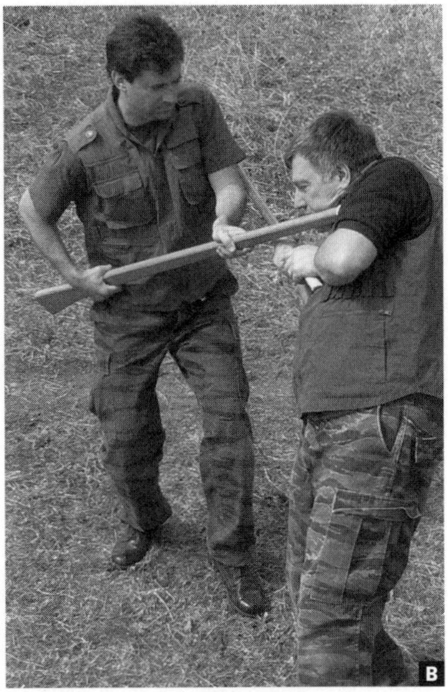

Figure 4-10b. Your opponent can easily recover and counterattack.

## Counterattack #2

In this situation you again block the attack with a raising sabre pose (Figure 4-11a). However, unlike counterattack #1, your opponent is so close you cannot step and slash.

If this occurs, strike him in the face with the pommel of your sabre (Figure 4-11b). The primary target area is the bones under the eyes next to the nose.

Hook his weapon and deliver the chop with your sabre (Figure 4-11c).

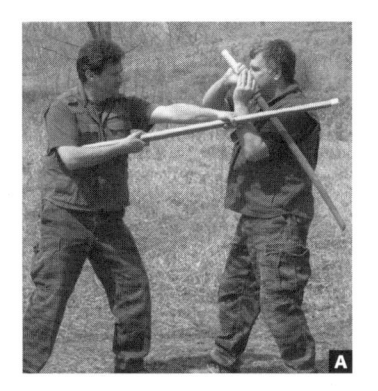

Figure 4-11a.

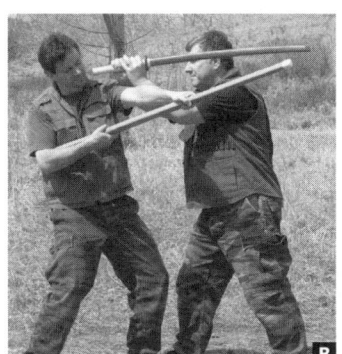

Figure 4-11b.

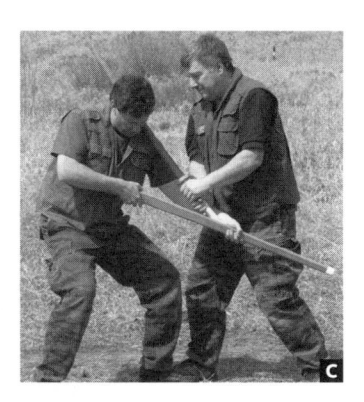

Figure 4-11c.

If your opponent moves backward, deliver a chop with your sabre. Or use a retreating step (see Section III on the *drilling sabre method*) and slash (Figure 4-12).

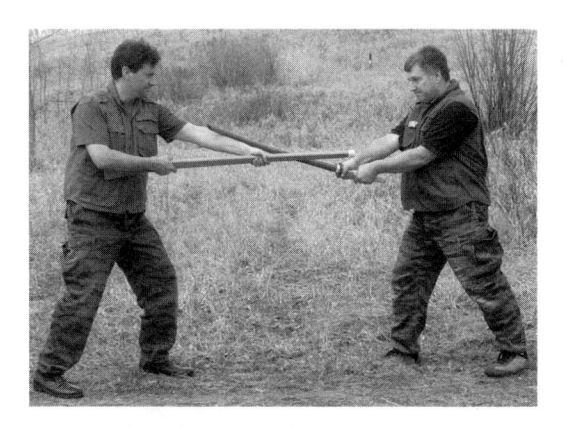

Figure 4-12. Use a retreating step and slash.

## ACTION #2: RIGHT POSITION

Stand with right foot forward. Imagine your opponent strikes or chops at the right side of your body. Quickly use your sabre to slash downward to the front right direction. Immediately assume the *upper hanging position* and follow through with a slash to the opponent's right side. Perform this strike in conjunction with a large step forward with the left foot.

In training, follow this sequence continuously, alternating left and right foot while moving forward.

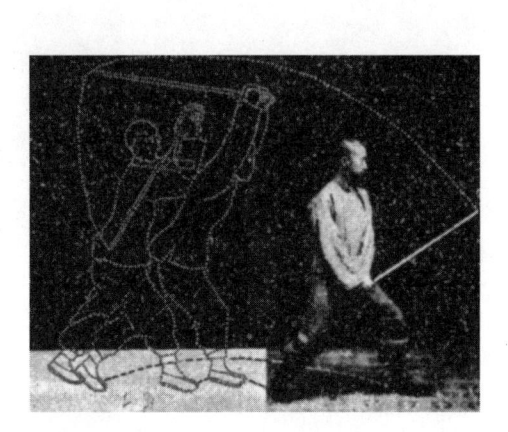

Figure 4-13.

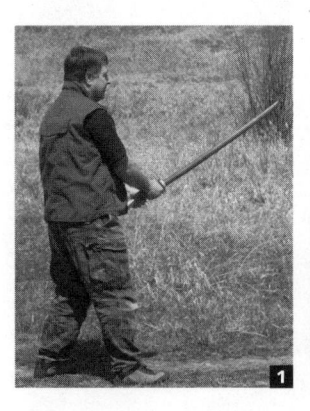

Figure 4-13m1.    Figure 4-13m2.    Figure 4-13m3.

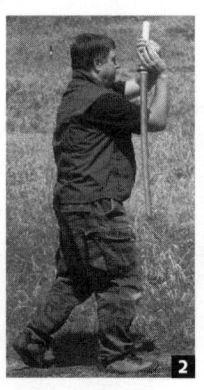

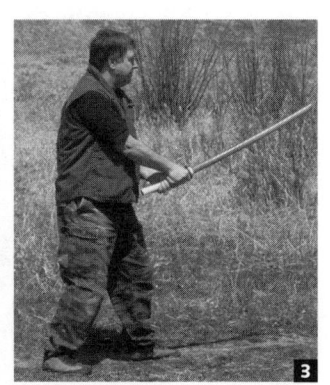

# EXPLANATION OF ACTION #2: CONSECUTIVE DOWNWARD SLASHES

In this sequence, Huang describes the use of two consecutive slashes as a means of countering an upper body attack. The first slash is executed without a block. This action could be used as:

- A feint or fake to throw the attacker off balance or cause him to react.
- A pre-emptive strike to the exposed side of his body (Figures 4-14a, 4-14b, and 4-14c). The object here is for you to cut him before he is able to make contact.

As well, training to deliver consecutive cuts serves two additional purposes:

- It teaches you to continue counterattacking until the opponent is finished. The assumption here is that your first slash was unsuccessful—you missed your target, your opponent's personal gear protected him, or your blow was not sufficient to incapacitate.
- It teaches you to deflect an attack to either side of your upper body, regardless of which foot is forward.

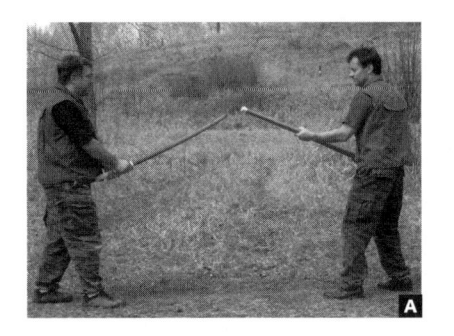

Figure 4-14a. Your opponent attacks (slightly out of range) with a straight thrust.

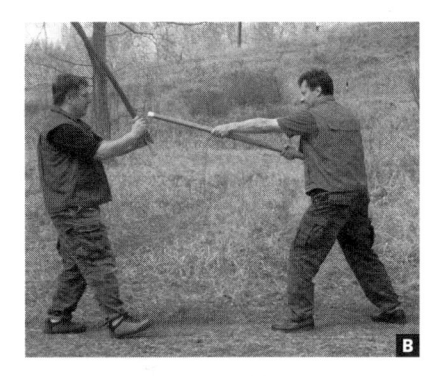

Figure 4-14b. You quickly raise your sabre.

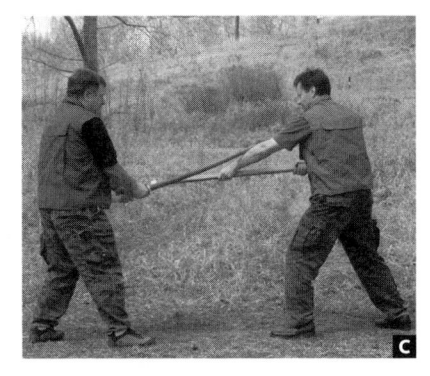

Figure 4-14c. Deliver a downward slash to his lead arm.

## FOOT POSITIONS AND TURNING

The majority of Huang's sabre instructions assume the left foot is forward or only describe the turning actions from the left-foot-forward position. There are two reasons for this.

1. Brevity. As was mentioned in the beginning of the book, Huang's text was written for instructors already versed in xingyi. They would be experienced enough to substitute "left" for "right" without any problem.
2. Convention. Huang was simply following a standardized method for training beginners. When novices first learned the basic stepping actions, they always turned from the left-foot-forward position in splitting, drilling, and crushing. In pounding and crossing, the turns were initially learned from the right-foot-forward position. Once the students were comfortable with turning in one direction, they learned how to turn from the other direction.

When I trained with Col. Chang in the early 1970s, he used this method of instruction. He also taught the orthodox or standardized (post–1928) moves in his xingyi style first and then went back and taught the older (pre–1928) variations.

# ACTION #3: TURNING AROUND

*"Stop . . . face the back . . . turn."*

When you hear the word "turn," note whether the left foot is forward. If it is, turn to the right. If right foot is in front, turn to the left.

Assuming your left foot is in front, push the sabre handle away from your body. This will cause the blade to face upward, with the point above your right shoulder and toward the back.

At the same time, take a small step backward with your right foot. As you turn your body, take a large step forward with your left foot and strike to the front of the opponent behind you. This complete action resembles the shape of a 360-degree cart wheel. *(That is, a circular movement resembling the wheel on a cart.)* You should end in *open position*.

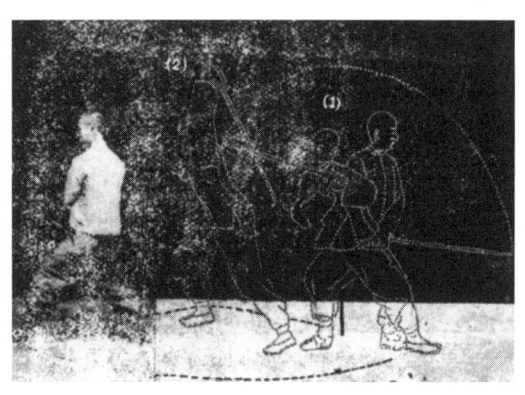

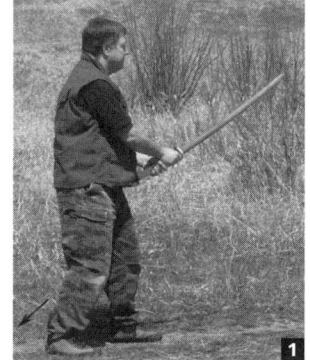

Figure 4-15.

Figure 4-15m1.

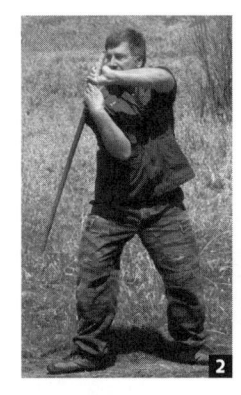

Figure 4-15m2.

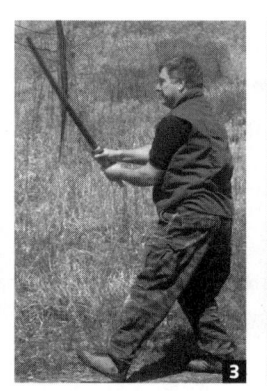

Figure 4-15m3.

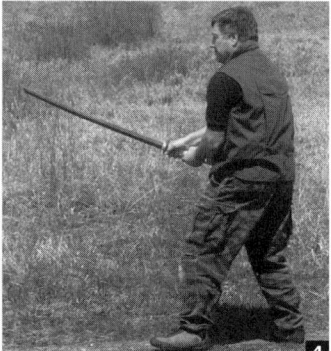

Figure 4-15m4.

## APPLICATION OF ACTION #3

As we see from Huang's description, this is a defense for an attack from behind. The assumption here is that the enemy will attack the largest and least mobile part of your body, your upper torso.

Because you can't see the level at which he is cutting or thrusting, you must automatically employ the raising sabre pose as you turn your head. Reinforced by your right shoulder, the blade protects the complete length of your upper body. As well, the blade is positioned for an immediate counterattack.

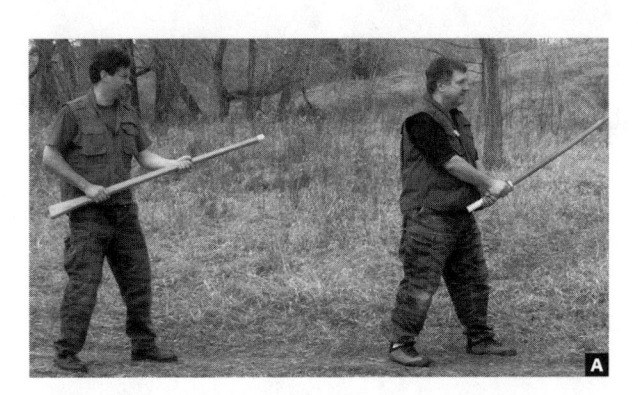

Figure 4-16a. Opponent attacks you from behind.

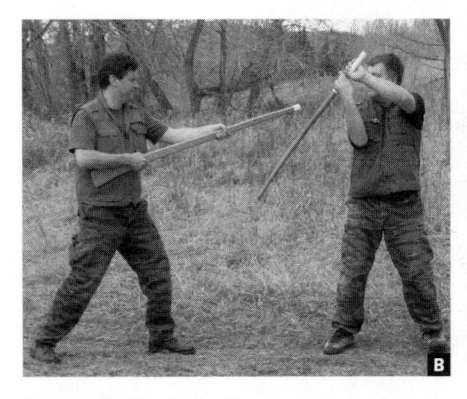

Figure 4-16b. As he thrusts, turn and block using raising sabre pose.

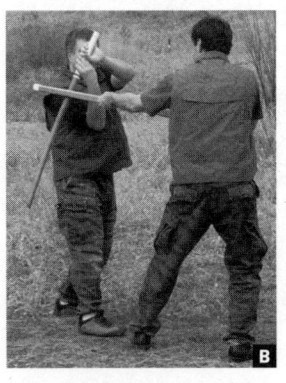

Figure 4-16br. Reverse angle showing how the sabre is carried alongside your body.

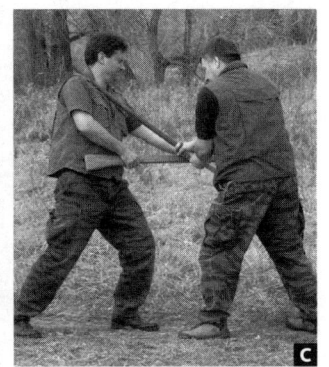

Figure 4-16c. Immediately slice him with your sabre.

# SECTION III: DRILLING SABRE METHOD

To make the transition from opening position to *drilling sabre position,* follow the orders:

*"Ready . . . drilling sabre . . . forward . . . go."*

**Action #1** (Figures 4-17 and 4-17m1 to 4-17m5 inclusive): Left Position *(attack against the left side)*. Imagine your opponent is chopping at the upper left side of your head. Employ your sabre vertically by turning the upper section *(front one-third of the blade)* in a *circular movement* [grinding wheel or grinding basin shape]. This action causes your opponent's weapon to be deflected and forced in the direction of the front left.

As you deflect, move your left foot slightly forward. Immediately step through with your right foot. (Use a large step.) Strike your opponent with a splitting action. Immediately retract the sabre by pulling your elbows in toward the body. Step backward with both feet. At the completion of this series of movements, your right foot will assume an open position.

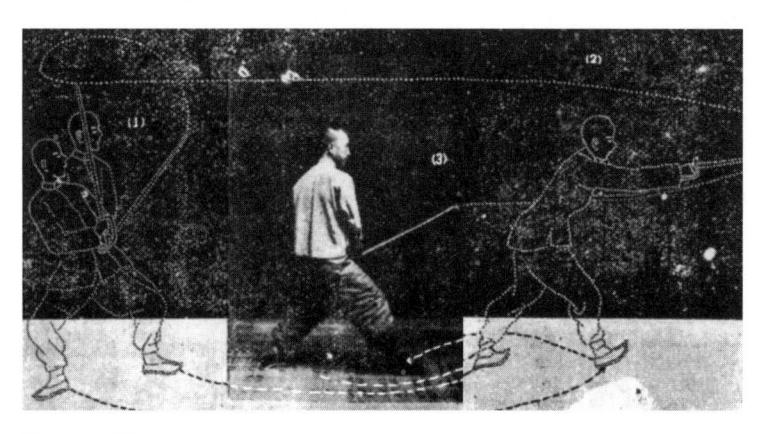

Figure 4-17.

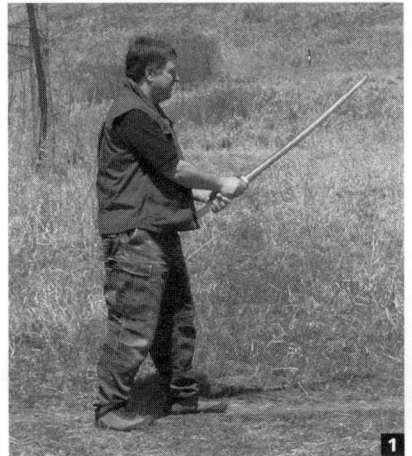

Figure 4-17m1.

Figure 4-17m2.

Figure 4-17m3.

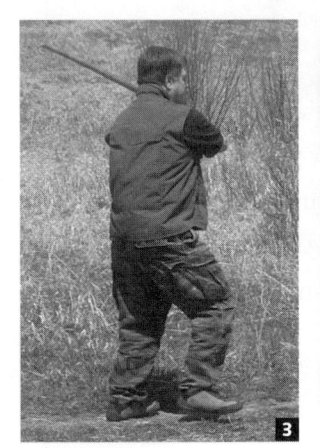

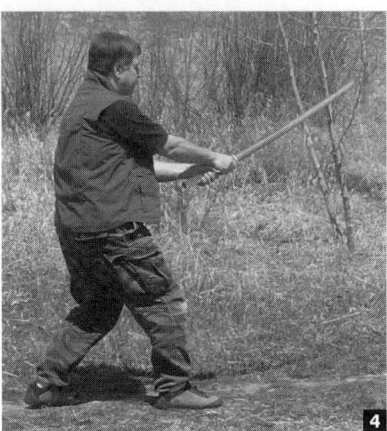

Figure 4-17m4.

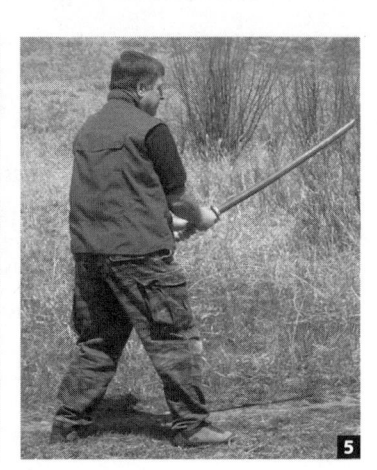

Figure 4-17m5.

## EXPLANATION OF CIRCULAR MOVEMENT

The circular movement described by Huang is a very subtle action. It consists of twisting the sabre as you pull both hands back to your side. The term "grinding wheel" or "grinding basin" refers to the circular action of the hands when using a pestle in a mortar or a stone hand grinder for grinding rice.

This circular movement with the front of the blade is primarily used when the opponent's attack is sudden, and you are caught off guard, or during an attack at close range. As a counter it is particularly useful when the opponent breaks the timing between stepping and striking.

In a bayonet attack, the turning action of your sabre delivers a quick chop to your opponent's lead hand and fingers (Figure 4-18a). Contact is made with the blade of your weapon.

If simply used as a block, the quick turning action of your blade (Figure 4-18b) causes the opponent's weapon to accelerate past your body.

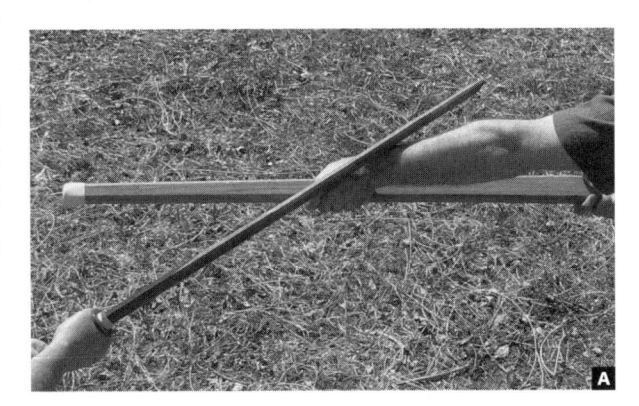

Figure 4-18a. Use the turning action to cut your opponent's hand.

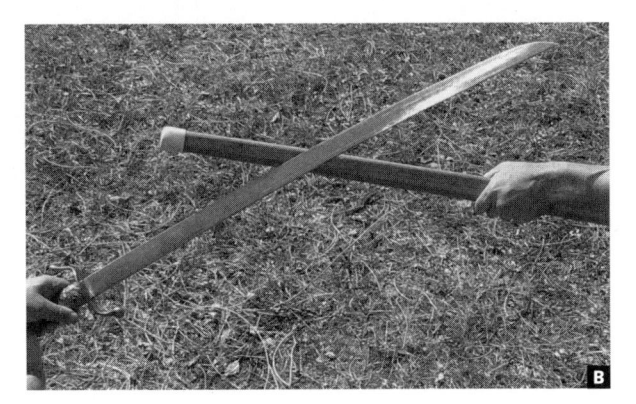

Figure 4-18b. The angle of the blade helps prevent it from being damaged.

## APPLICATION OF ACTION #1

Your opponent attacks the left side of your head (Figure 4-19a).

Use the circular motion to deflect his weapon (Figure 4-19b).

Step through with your right foot and strike (Figure 4-19c).

If the attacker is slightly out of range but closes distance (Figure 4-19d), deflect and step back (Figure 4-19e).

Slash his lead arm or hand (Figure 4-19f).

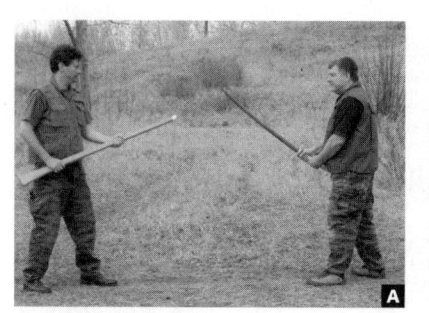

Figure 4-19a.

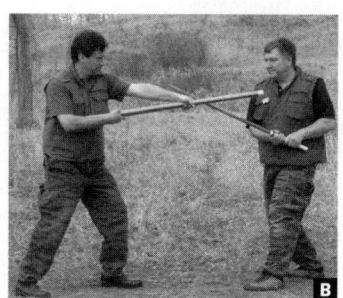

Figure 4-19b.

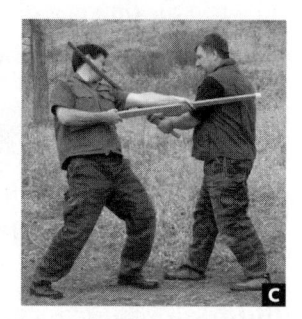

Figure 4-19c.

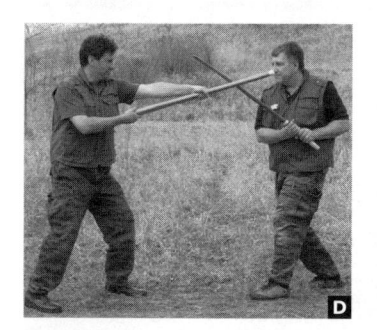

Figure 4-19d.

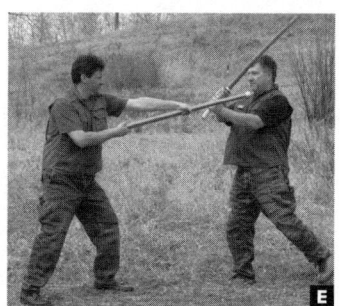

Figure 4-19e.

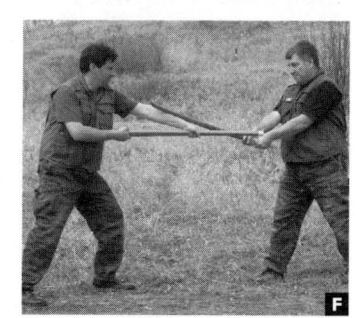

Figure 4-19f.

# ACTION #2: RIGHT POSITION

*(This action is for defending against attack against your right side while in right forward stance.)* Imagine your opponent chops at the upper right side of your head. Use the circular movement to deflect his weapon to the right front direction, away from your body. As you deflect, take a small step with your right foot. Immediately take a large step forward and through with the left foot. As you step, chop to your opponent's right side.

Quickly pull the sabre back, as in Action #1, and step backward with both feet. You should now be in an open position with left foot forward.

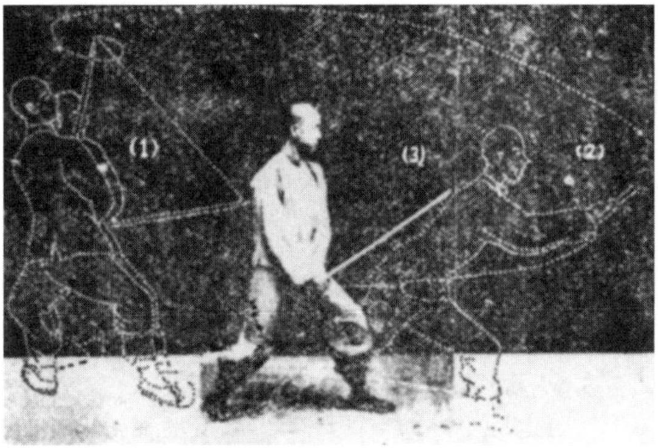

Figure 4-20.

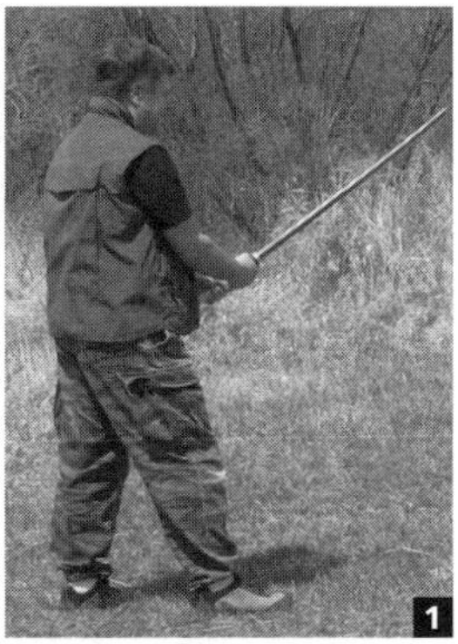

Figure 4-20m1.

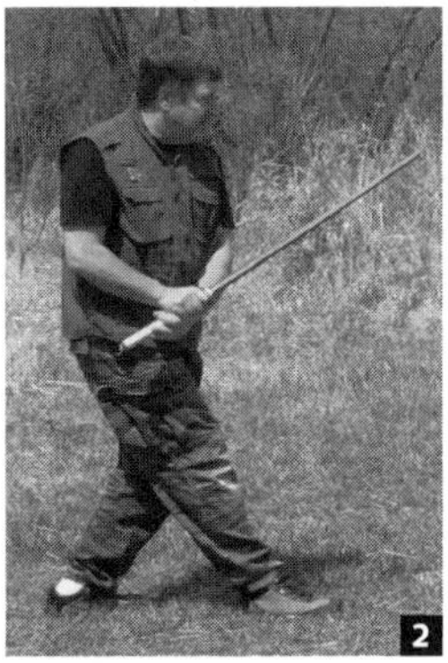

Figure 4-20m2.

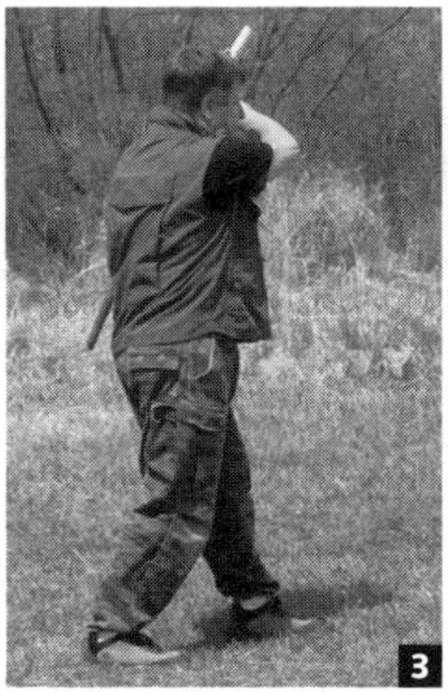

Figure 4-20m3.

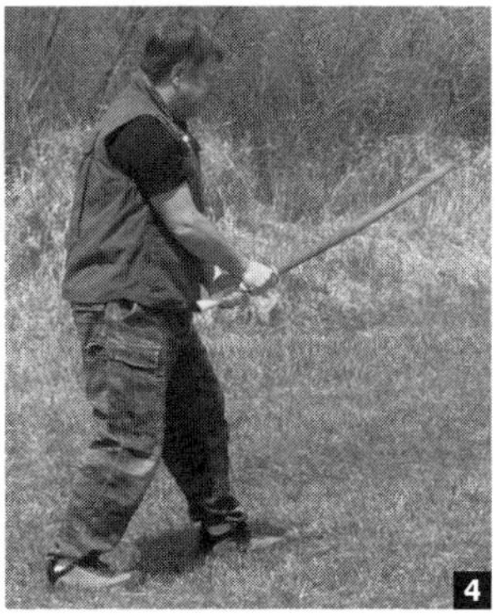

Figure 4-20m4.

## ACTION #3

To turn around from drilling sabre forward position, follow the orders:

*"Stop . . . to the back . . . turn."*

Imagine your opponent is trying to strike at you from behind. Grasp the sabre with both hands and counter the strike with a downward slash. Your defensive action begins with hands positioned near your right ear. Turn blade using the circular motion. As you turn the blade, step forward with the left foot and quickly cut the opponent.

To recover, pull both your sabre and feet back to the ready position.

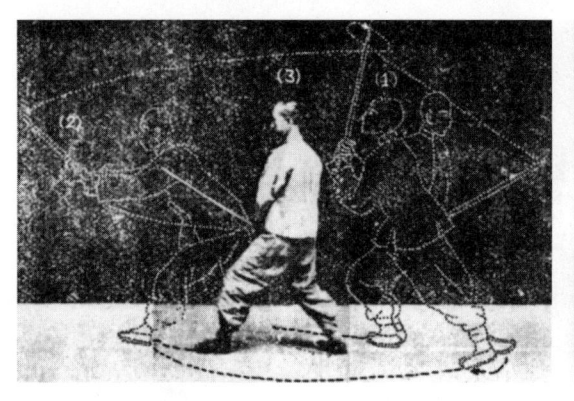

Figure 4-21.

Figure 4-21m1.

Figure 4-21m2.

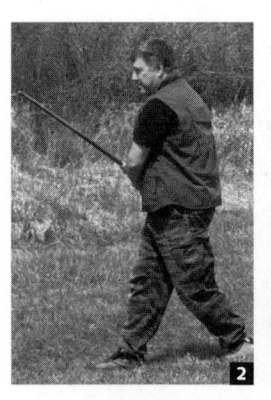

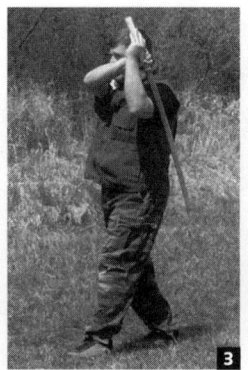

Figure 4-21m3.

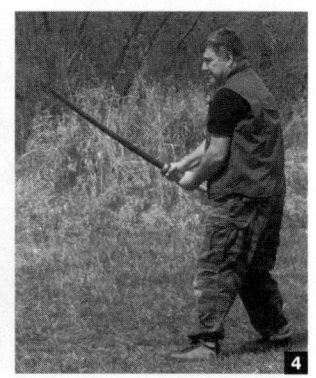

Figure 4-21m4.

# SECTION IV: CRUSHING SABRE METHOD

To make the transition from opening position to *crushing sabre position*, follow the orders:

*"Ready . . . crushing sabre . . . forward . . . go."*

**Action #1** (Figures 4-22 and 4-22m1 to 4-22m4 inclusive): Left Position. Imagine your opponent thrusts at your stomach. Use the tip of your sabre (in the upper right position) to make a small circle. Move your blade downward and deflect the opponent's weapon. Immediately counterattack with a straight thrust to the opponent's midsection.

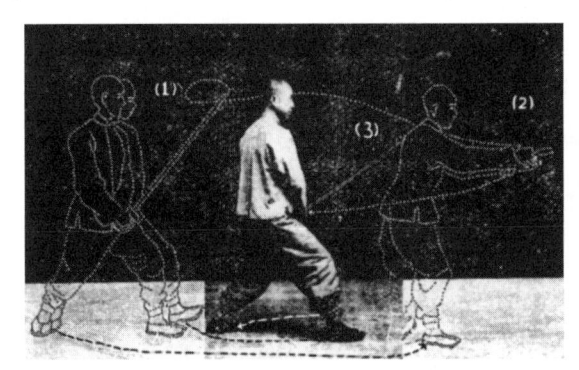

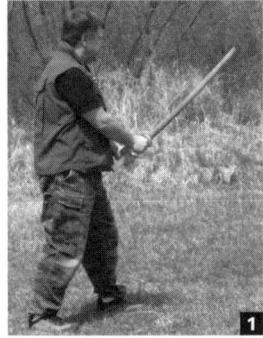

Figure 4-22.

Figure 4-22m1.

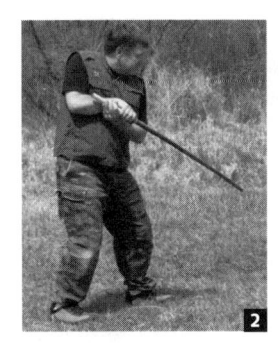

Figure 4-22m2.

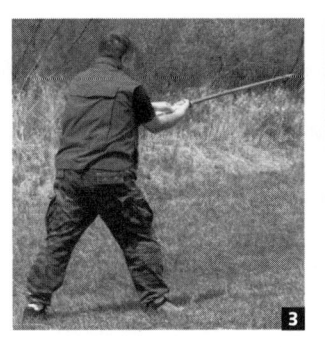

Figure 4-22m3.

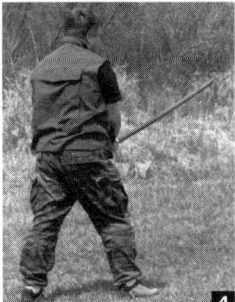

Figure 4-22m4.

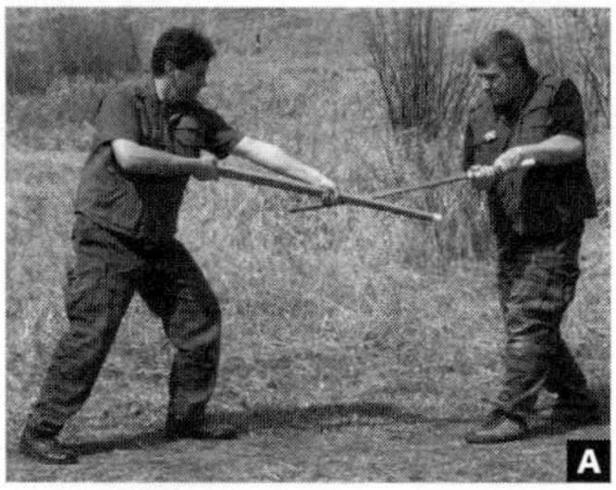

Figure 4-23a.

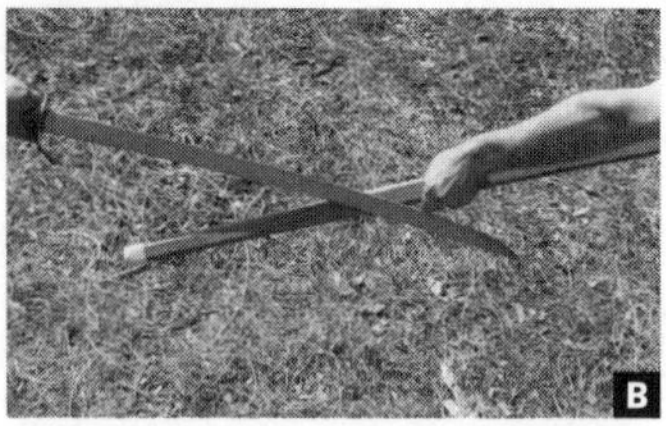

Figure 4-23b.

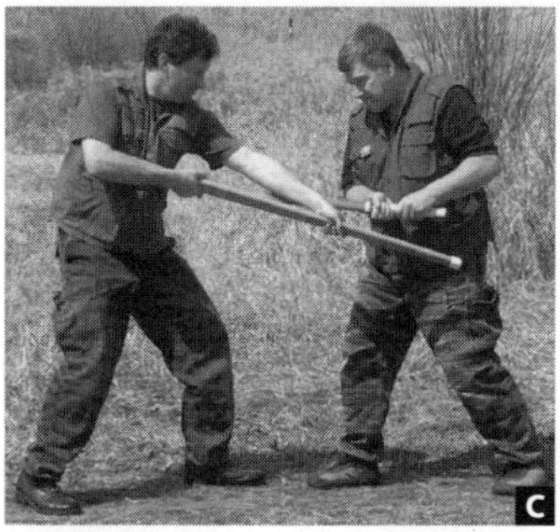

Figure 4-23c.

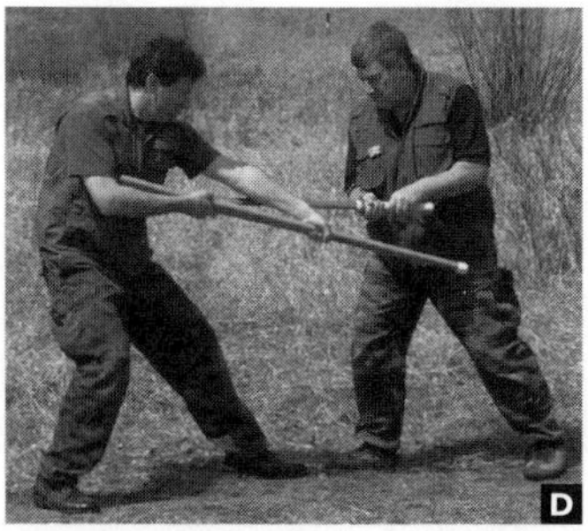

Figure 4-23d.

As you counterattack, step forward (slightly) with your left foot. Immediately follow this with a large step (approximately 3 feet) with the right foot. Right foot lands in front of left foot. As your right foot comes to rest, pull the sabre back to the ready position. Right foot remains forward.

## APPLICATION OF ACTION #1

Note that this example shows an alternative method of stepping. As your opponent thrusts, drop the tip of your blade and slice his lead hand (Figure 4-23a). Rotate the blade so it cuts across and up. This motion will allow you to simultaneously cut his hand and deflect his weapon with the flat of your blade. Once again this prevents you from damaging the cutting edge of your sabre (Figure 4-23b).

Move in, slicing his arm and keeping your blade close to his weapon (Figure 4-23c).

Stab him in the stomach or groin (Figure 4-23d).

# ACTION #2

If your right side is forward, make a circle by moving your sabre's tip from the upper left position (as described in Action #1). Move your right foot slightly forward. Take a large step forward and through with your left foot. Left foot should land in front of right foot. (This step is approximately 3 feet in length.) Immediately follow this step with either a cut to the opponent's wrist or a thrust to his stomach. Quickly retract the sabre and return to the ready position. Left foot remains in front.

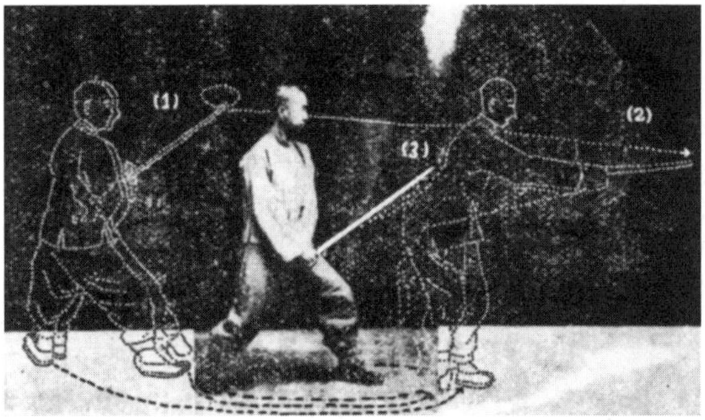

Figure 4-24.

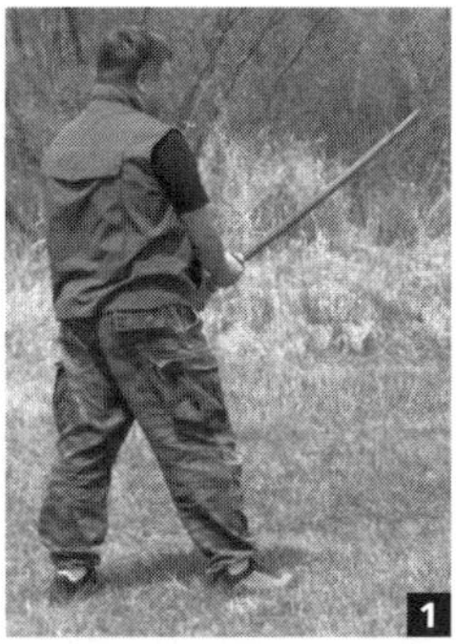

Figure 4-24m1.

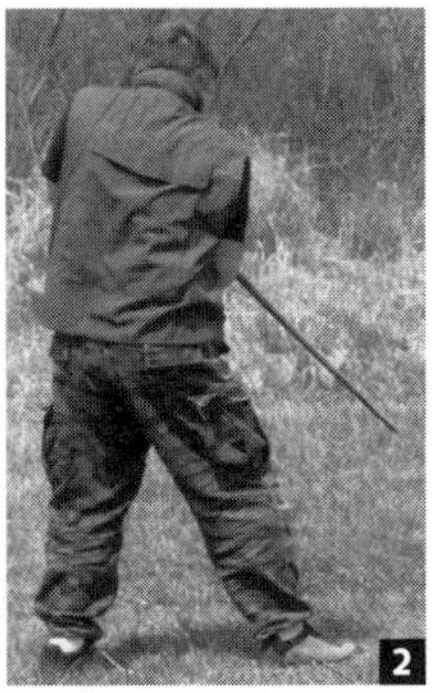

Figure 4-24m2.

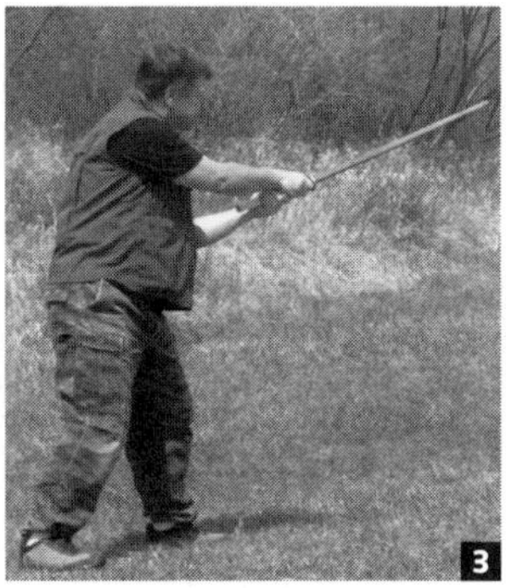

Figure 4-24m3.

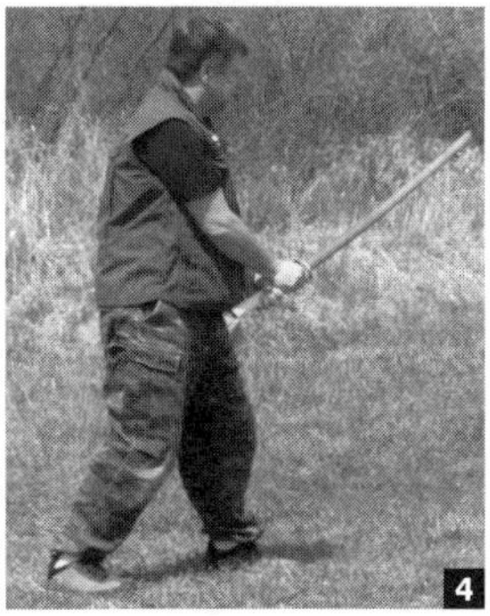

Figure 4-24m4.

## ACTION #3

To turn around from crushing sabre forward position, follow the orders:

*"Stop . . . face the back . . . turn."*

If your left foot is forward when the order is heard, move the tip of your sabre downward. Pull both hands back to the right side of the body. At the same time, raise your right foot and *wrap the hanging half circle shape*. Horizontally turn [flip] the sabre and execute a scissor step movement.

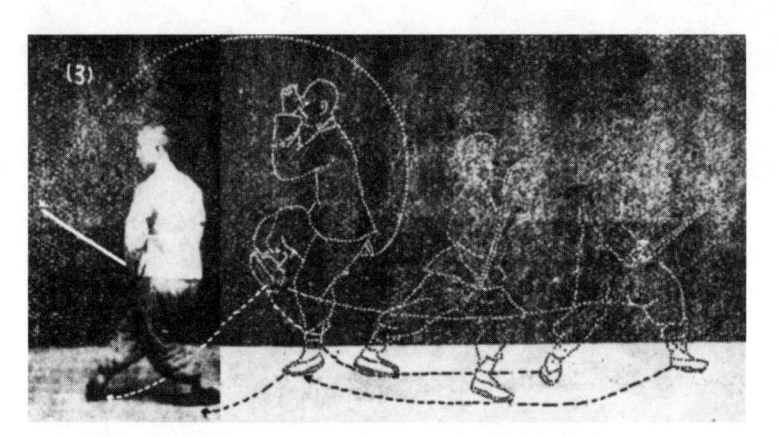

Figure 4-25.

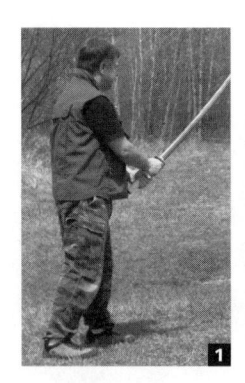

Figure 4-25m1.

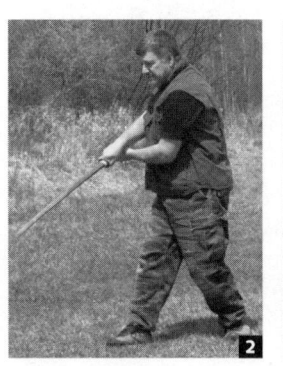

Figure 4-25m2.

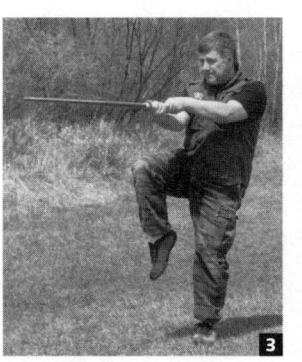

Figure 4-25m3.

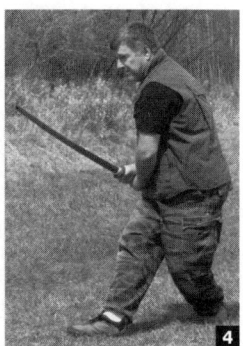

Figure 4-25m4.

# SECTION V: POUNDING SABRE METHOD

To make the transition from holding sabre position to *pounding sabre position*, follow the orders:

*"Ready . . . pounding sabre . . . forward . . . go."*

**Action#1** (Figures 4-26 and 4-26m1, 4-26m2, and 4-26m3): Imagine your opponent chops to the left side of your body. In this instance it does not matter if the action is to the upper or lower part. Immediately use both hands to raise the sabre's handle toward the ceiling. The back

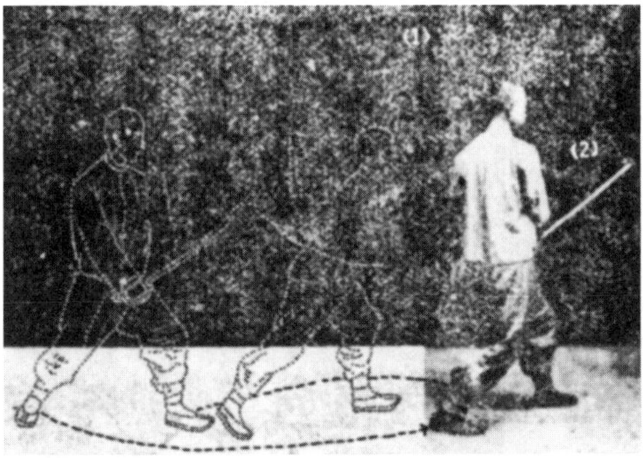

Figure 4-26.

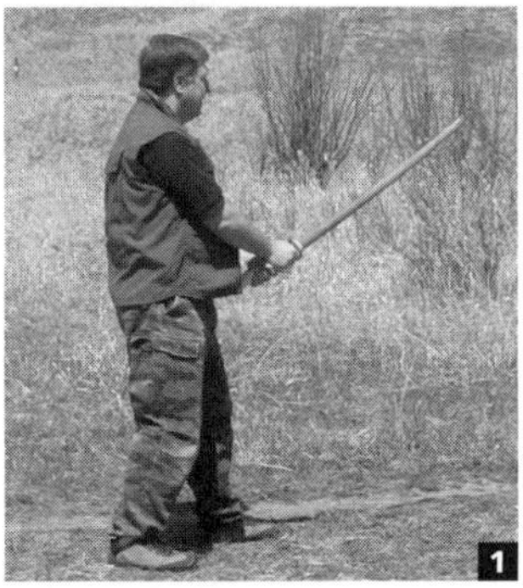

Figure 4-26m1. 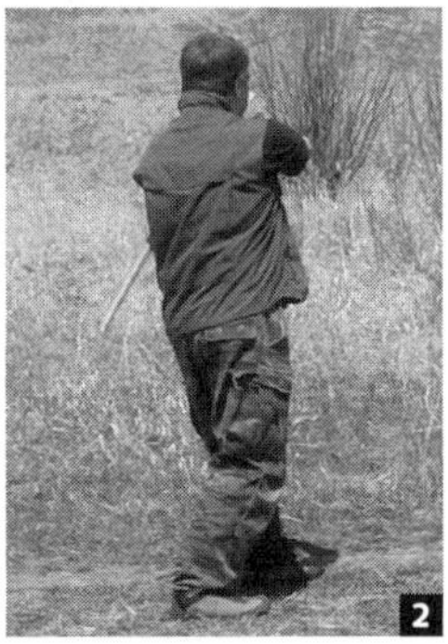　　　Figure 4-26m2. 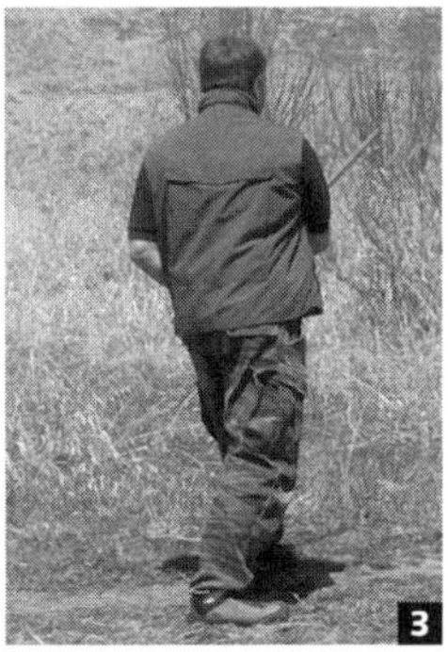　　　Figure 4-26m3.

side of your sabre should touch your left shoulder. Use *ging (strength or force)* to deflect the opponent's weapon to your left side. At the same time, strike the opponent's shoulder. The sabre and left foot should form a triangle as in the *pounding fist step*.

## FIRST APPLICATION OF ACTION #1 (CLOSE-RANGE ATTACK)

Your opponent attempts a close-range slash (Figure 4-27a).

You immediately counter by raising your sabre and cutting his wrists (Figure 4-27b).

Stepping through the center line of his body (between his legs) you push the blade against his neck (Figure 4-27c).

Continue stepping as you draw the blade and cut (Figure 4-27d).

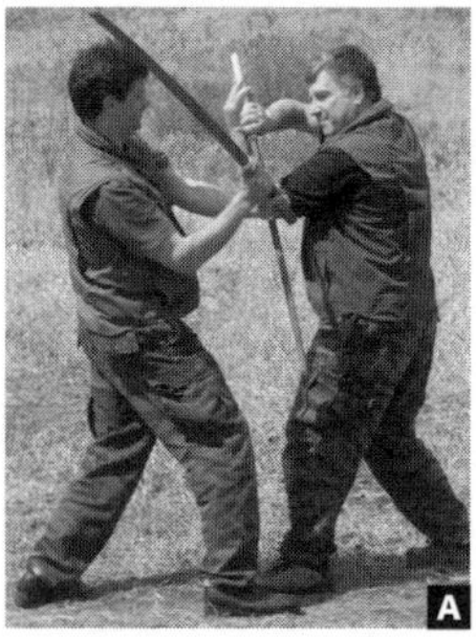

Figure 3-27a. 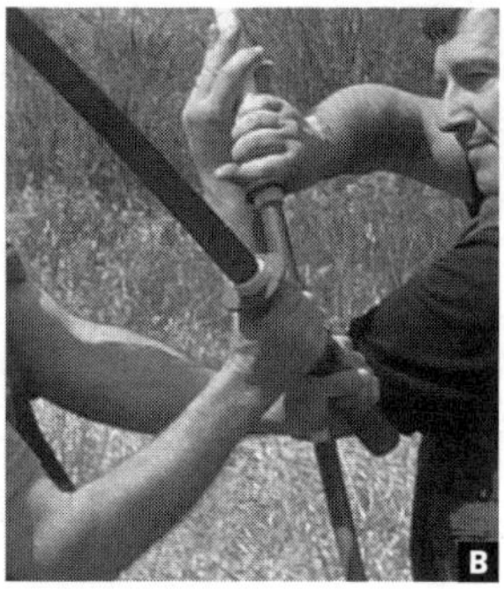   Figure 3-27b. 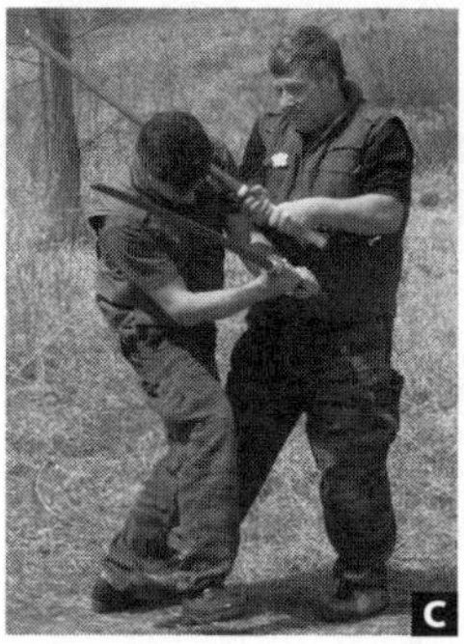   Figure 3-27c. 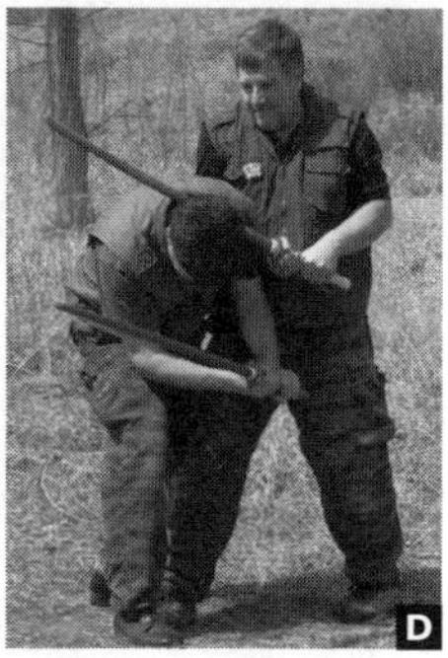   Figure 3-27d.

Chapter Four  **131**

# SECOND APPLICATION OF ACTION #1 (LONG-RANGE ATTACK)

As your opponent attempts to slash, use a diagonal step through the center line of his body to close distance (Figure 4-28a).

Use your blade to cover the left side of your body (Figure 4-28b).

Counter with a quick slash to his neck (Figure 4-28c).

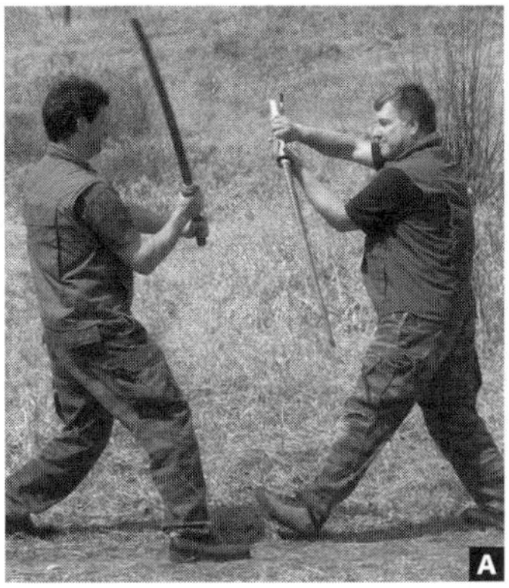

Figure 2-28a.

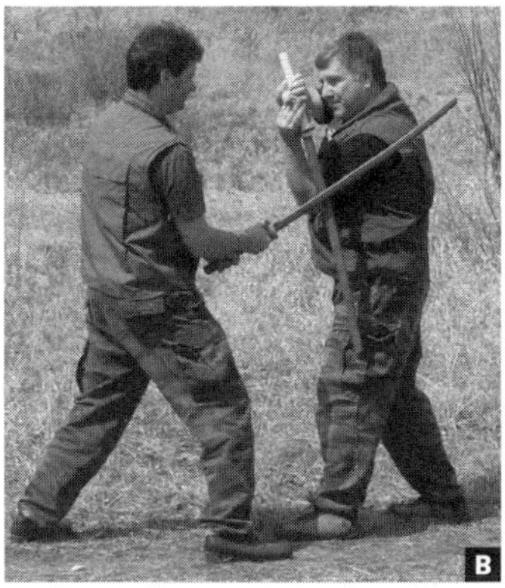

Figure 2-28b.

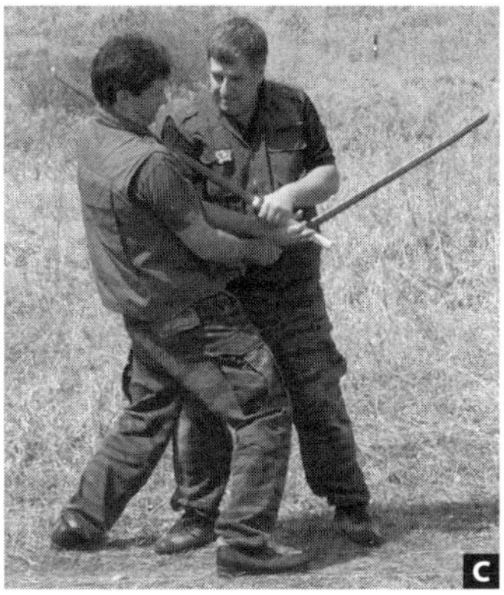

Figure 2-28c.

## ACTION #2

Stand in the right side ready position. Imagine your opponent thrusts or chops to the right side. Using the form described above, allow the back of the blade to touch your right shoulder. Immediately deflect the opponent's blade. Follow with a strike to your opponent's right side. This movement is done so that your right foot and sabre form the *pounding fist triangle*. The feet should end approximately 1 foot apart.

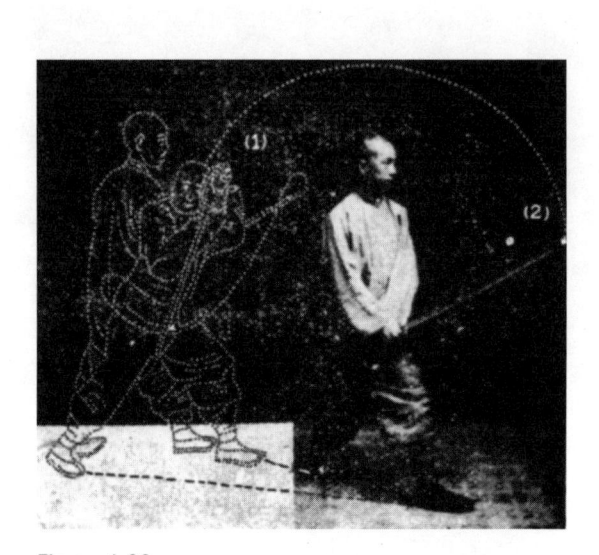

Figure 4-29.

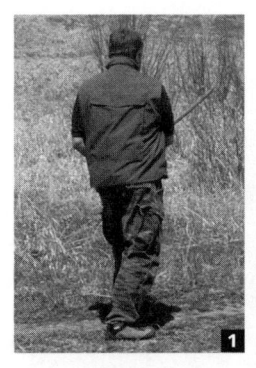

Figure 4-29m1.   Figure 4-29m2.   Figure 4-29m3.

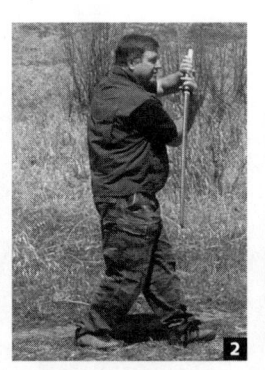

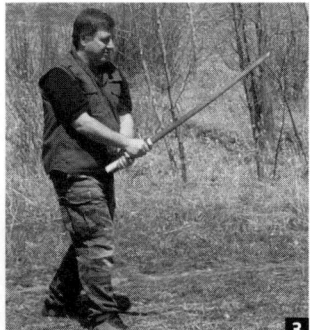

## APPLICATION OF ACTION #2

Your opponent faces you (Figure 4-30a).

He steps and attempts to slash your right side. You step diagonally, block, and cut his wrists (Figure 4-30b).

Immediately flip your sabre and follow with a downward slash to your opponent's right side (Figure 4-30c). (Note: In this photo the defender steps through to apply additional force to his cut.)

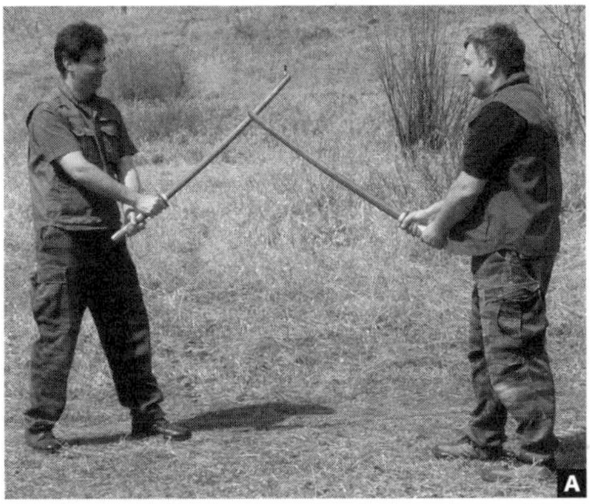

Figure 4-30a.

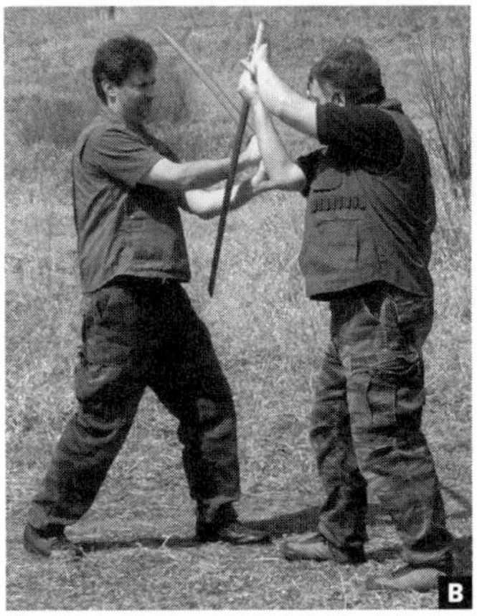

Figure 4-30b.

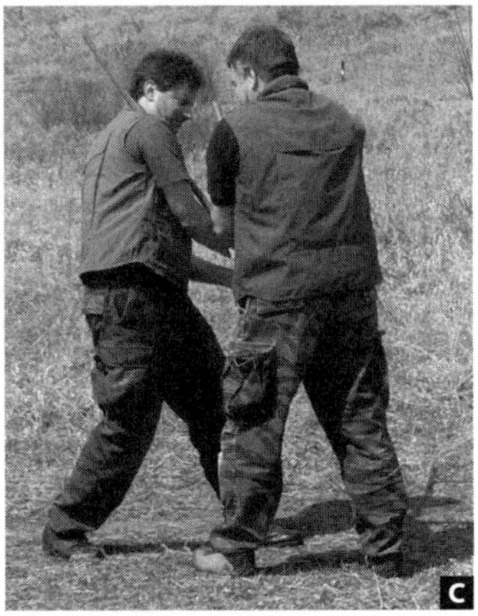

Figure 4-30c.

## ACTION #3

To turn around from forward position, follow the orders:

*"Stop . . . to the back . . . turn."*

When you hear the word "turn," turn to the left. As you complete the turn, execute a splitting movement to the back right direction. During this turn it is important to keep the handle of the sabre pointing upward to deflect the opponent's weapon.

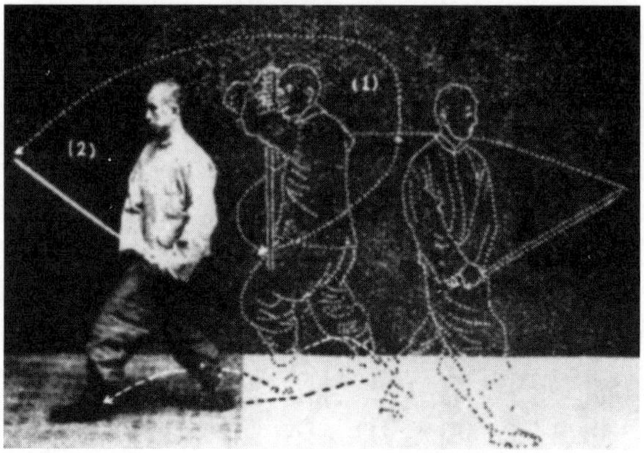

Figure 4-31.

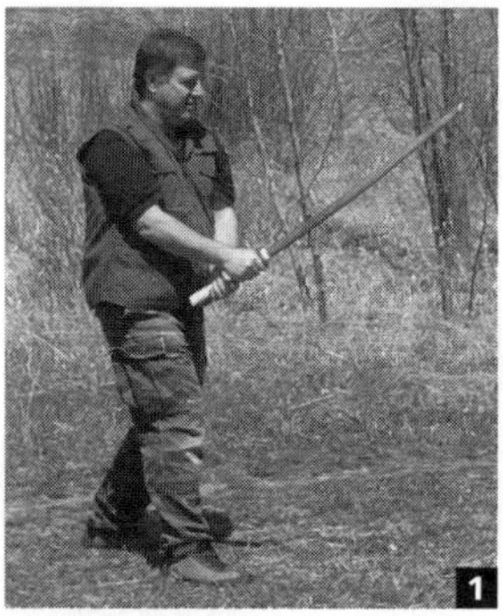

Figure 4-31m1. 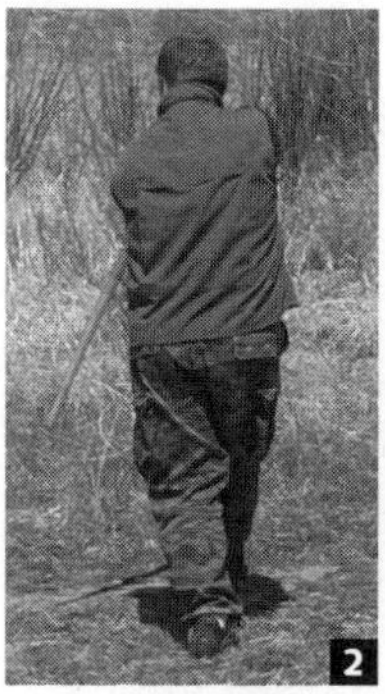   Figure 4-31m2. 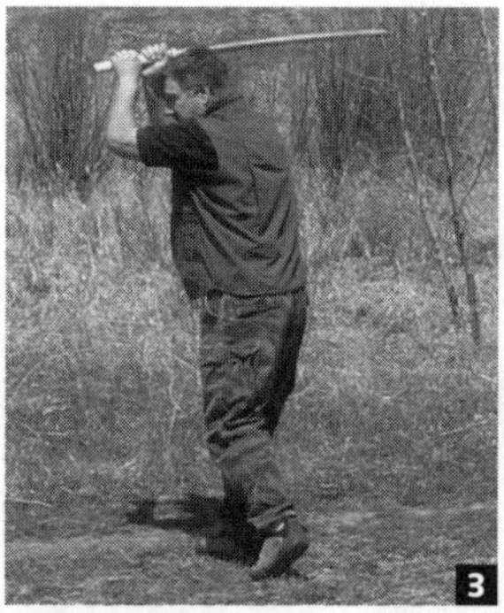   Figure 4-31m3. 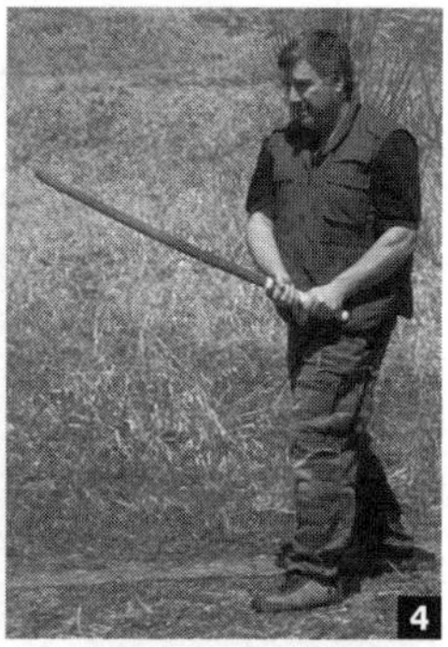   Figure 4-31m4.

# SECTION VI: CROSSING SABRE METHOD

To make the transition from holding sabre position to the *crossing sabre position*, follow the orders:

*"Ready . . . crossing sabre . . . forward . . . go."*

**Action #1** (Figure 4-32 and 4-32m1 to 4-32m6 inclusive): Imagine your opponent thrusts to your left shoulder. Move the tip of your sabre to your left side and deliver a horizontal strike to his weapon. This should be done in such a manner that his weapon becomes positioned above your weapon. Employ the circular movement to horizontally cut your opponent's waist. Continue the horizontal movement until your sabre and front left foot fall in a straight line. This is the same as crossing or horizontal step.

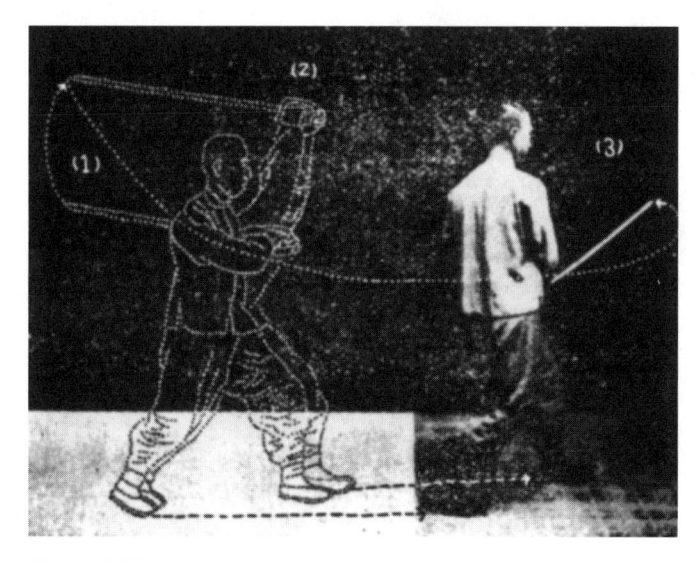

Figure 4-32.

Figure 4-32m1.

Figure 4-32m2.

Figure 4-32m3.

Figure 4-32m4.

Figure 4-32m5.

Figure 4-32m6.

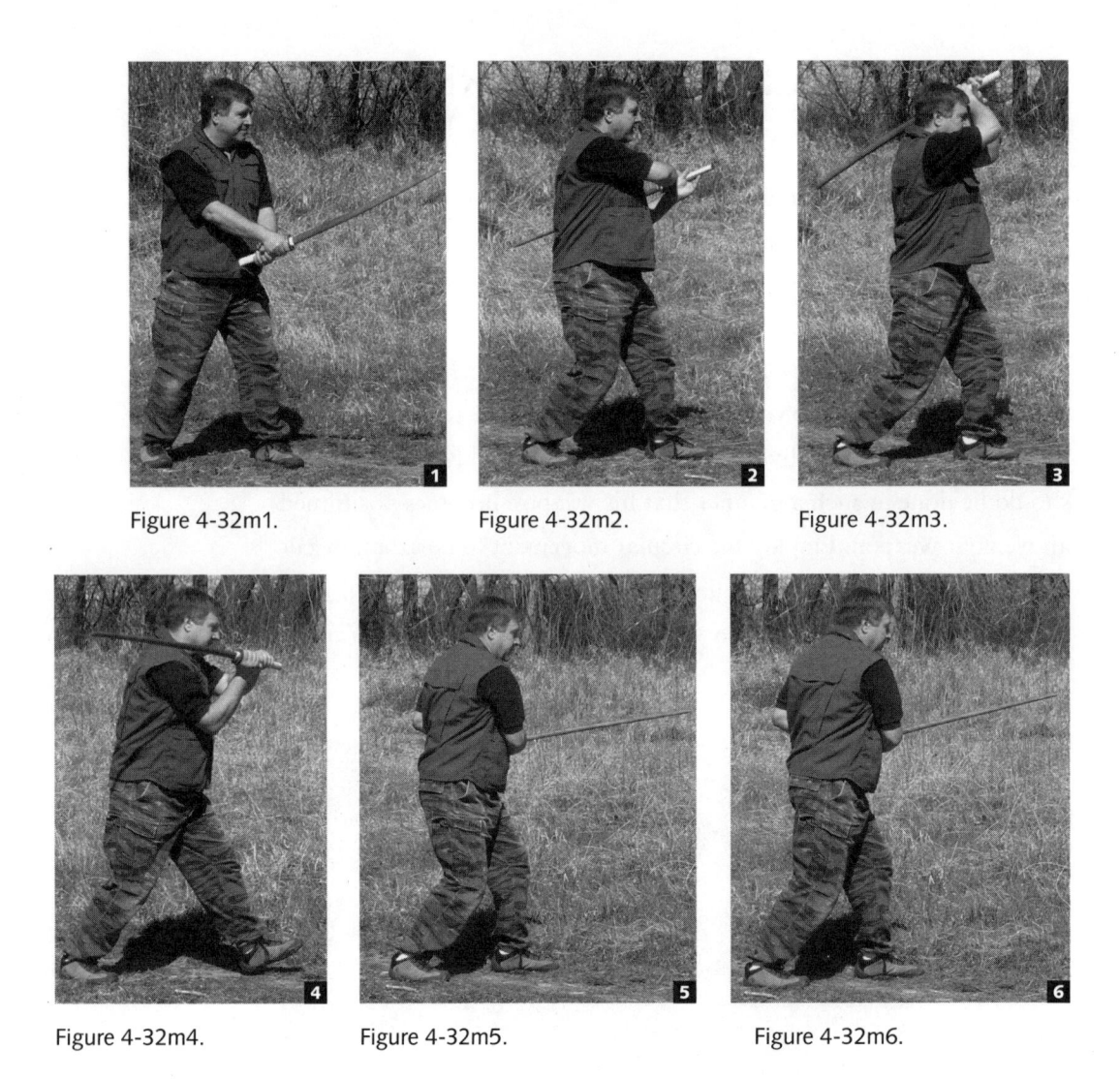

*(In Chinese the character for "horizontal" does not necessarily mean perfectly parallel to the ground. The object, in this case the blade, can be at an angle. As well, "horizontal" in Huang's usage also means that the blade is flat [not vertical, or with cutting edge down].)*

Chapter Four

## APPLICATION OF ACTION #1

Your opponent attacks your left shoulder with a high thrust. As you step, counter with a horizontal deflection (Figure 4-33a).

Continue the circular action with your sabre (Figure 4-33b).

Deliver a downward strike to your opponent's left side (Figure 4-33c).

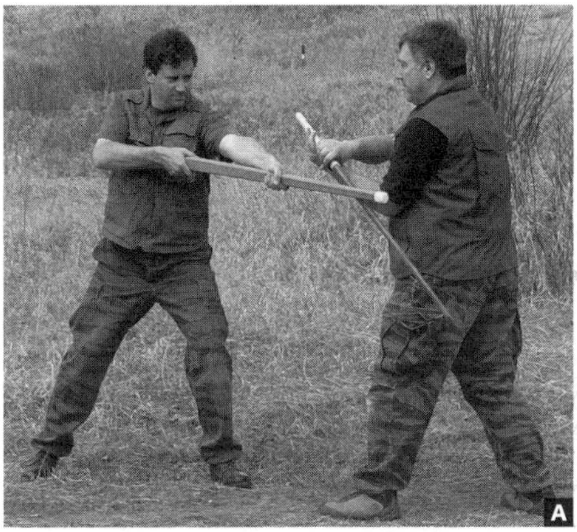

Figure 4-33a.

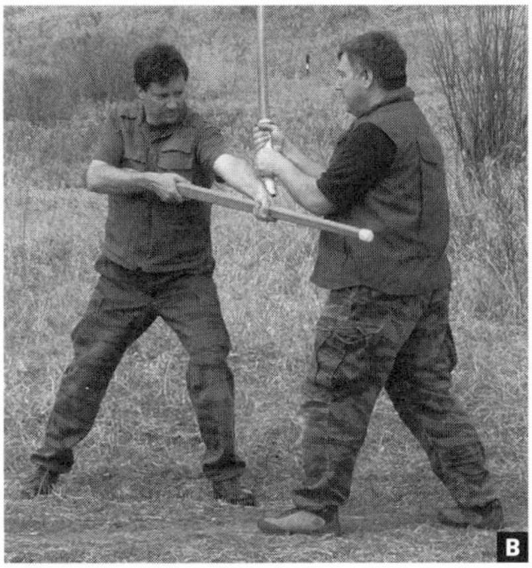

Figure 4-33b.

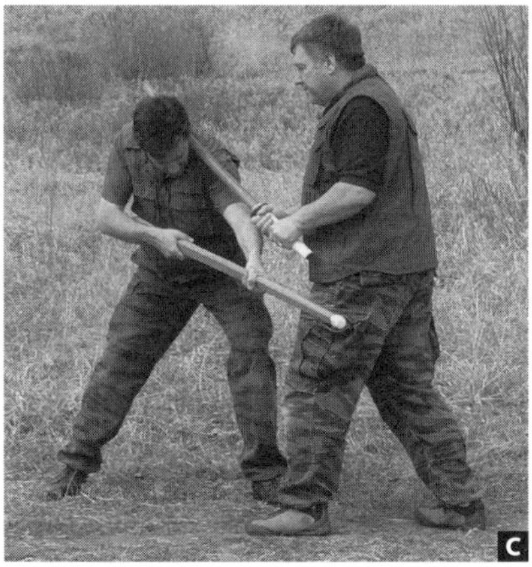

Figure 4-33c.

## ACTION #2

Imagine your opponent is attacking your right side. Utilize the movement described above, but strike horizontally to the right and cut your opponent's waist. *(That is, use the same sequence of moves as in Action #1, only perform them on the right side.)* This movement should end with the sabre and right foot in alignment.

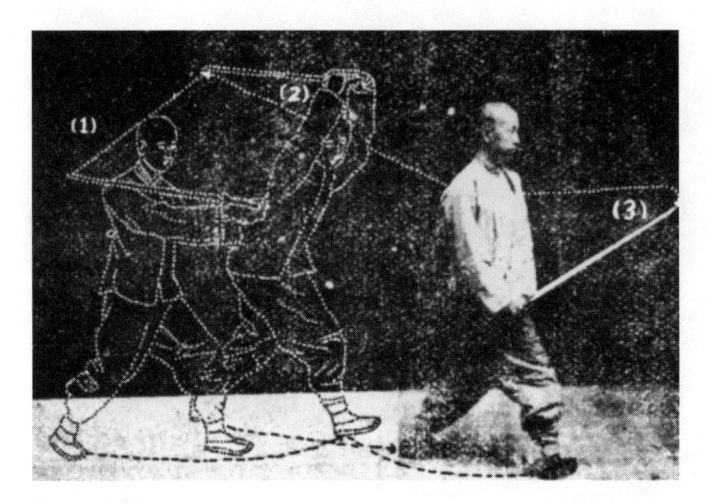

Figure 4-34.

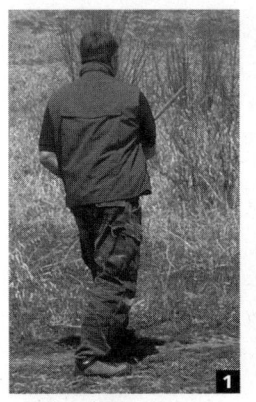

Figure 4-34m1.  Figure 4-34m2.  Figure 4-34m3.

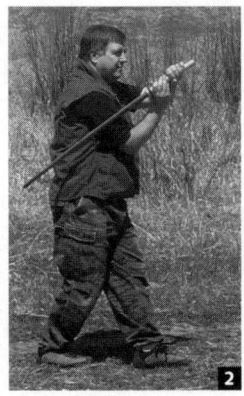

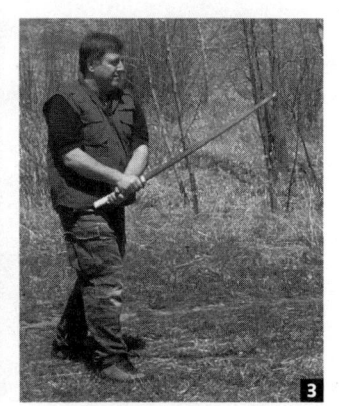

# ACTION #3

To turn around from forward position, follow the orders:

*"Stop . . . to the back . . . turn."*

When you hear the order and assuming your right foot is forward, immediately turn to the left. (If left foot is forward, turn to the right.) As you turn, strike diagonally to the back, left direction, using the flat or horizontal blade. After you complete the diagonal left strike, continue to strike to the left front direction. Your sabre and left front foot should align.

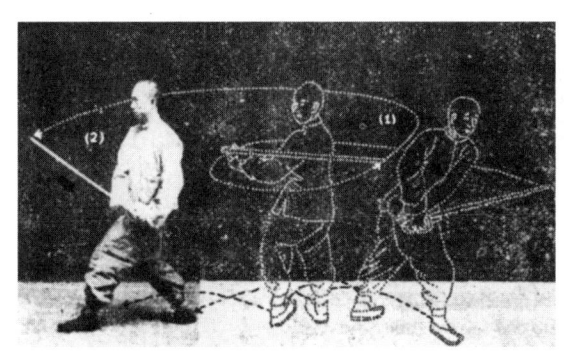

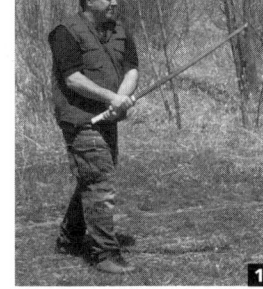

Figure 4-35.

Figure 4-35m1.

Figure 4-35m2.

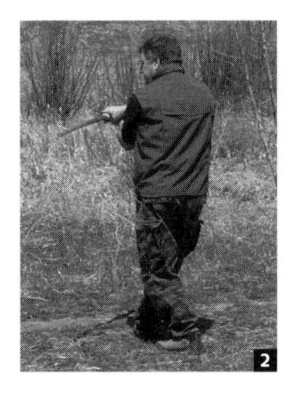

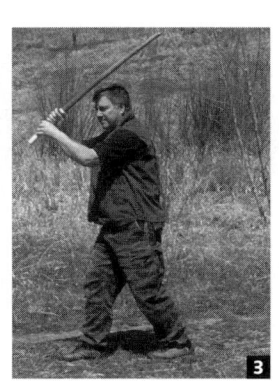

Figure 4-35m3.

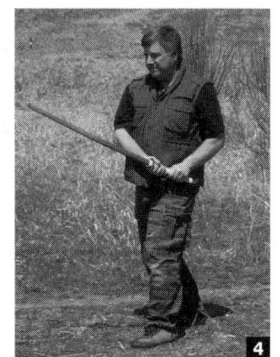

Figure 4-35m4.

# XINGYI TERMS
## IN ENGLISH AND CHINESE

### Chapter 1

| | |
|---|---|
| Five Elements | 五行 |
| Metal | 金 |
| Wood | 木 |
| Water | 水 |
| Fire | 火 |
| Earth | 土 |
| Assisting Theory | 相生之道 |
| Hindering Theory | 相剋之義 |
| Crushing Fist | 弸拳 |
| Drilling Fist | 鑽拳 |
| Splitting Fist | 劈拳 |
| Pounding or Exploding Fist | 炮拳 |
| Crossing or Horizontal Fist | 橫拳 |
| Linking Fist Form | 連環拳 |
| Qi (air; energy) | 氣 |
| Eight Rules or Secrets | 八字訣 |
| Nine Songs of the Beginning Position | 開式九歌 |

# Xingyi Terms

**Chapter 2**

| | |
|---|---|
| Standing Position | 立正姿勢 |
| Right Half Turn Position | 半面向右轉姿勢 |
| Opening Position | 開式勢 |
| Route Illustration | 路線圖說 |
| Turning Around | 向後轉 |
| Pici (Cut and Slash) | 劈刺 |

**Chapter 3**

| | |
|---|---|
| Standing at Attention | 立正姿勢 |
| Ready Position | 預備姿勢 |
| Step Thrust Position | 步刺 |
| Horizontal Blade Position | 端平鎗 |
| Crushing Rifle Position | 弸鎗勢 |
| Wiping Motion | 迎撥 |
| Ti Guai Lei Position | 鐵拐子勢 |
| Smooth Style Pounding Rifle | 順式炮鎗 |
| Crushing Style Stance | 弸鎗式 |
| Stepping Backward Stance | 倒踏步 |
| Scissor Hip (Cross) Stance | 剪子股式 |
| Back Step Chop Rifle | 退步劈鎗 |
| Smooth Style Crushing Rifle | 順式弸鎗 |
| Yang Palm | 陽掌 |
| Yin Palm | 陰掌 |
| Exploding Rifle Stance | 炮鎗式 |
| Chop Rifle Step | 劈鎗式 |

Ba (numeral 8) Shape 八字形
Backward Step Horizontal Rifle 退步橫鎗
Drilling Rifle Method 鑽鎗式
Face the Wind; Slash; Nick 迎風劃挑
Detach (or Escape) Changing (or Exchanging) Shadow 脫身換影

## Chapter 4

Raising Sabre Pose 舉刀勢
Holding Sabre Pose 持刀勢
Hidden Sword Position 藏刀式
Parting the Horse's Mane 分鬃式
Grinding Wheel or Grinding Basin Shape 磨盤形
Upper Hanging Position 上掛

# XINGYI LINEAGE OF DENNIS ROVERE

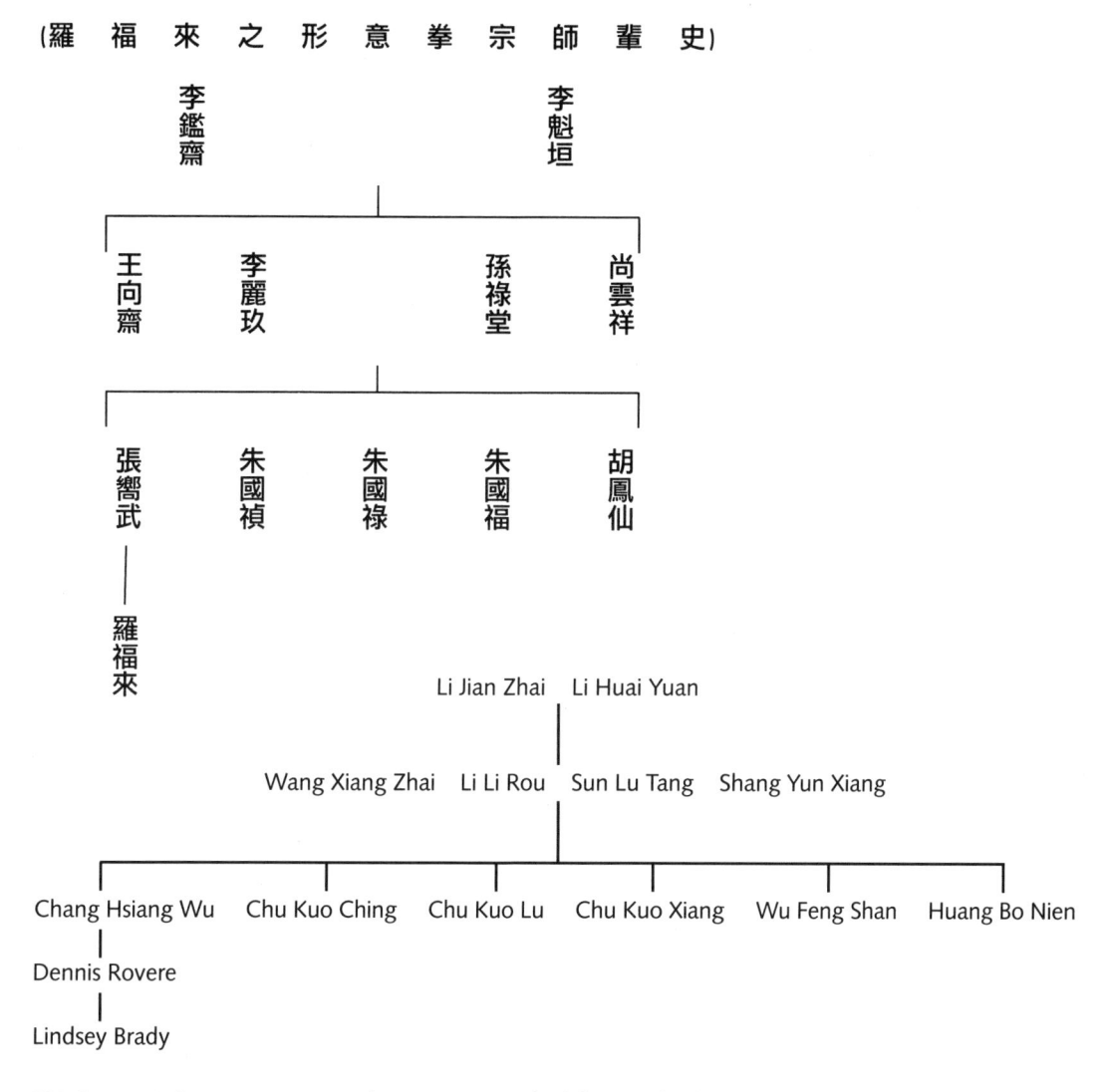

(羅福來之形意拳宗師輩史)

李鑑齋　　　　　　　李魁垣

王向齋　李麗玖　　孫祿堂　尚雲祥

張嚮武　朱國禎　朱國祿　朱國福　胡鳳仙

羅福來

```
                    Li Jian Zhai    Li Huai Yuan
                           |
    Wang Xiang Zhai    Li Li Rou   Sun Lu Tang    Shang Yun Xiang

Chang Hsiang Wu   Chu Kuo Ching   Chu Kuo Lu   Chu Kuo Xiang   Wu Feng Shan   Huang Bo Nien
      |
Dennis Rovere
      |
Lindsey Brady
```

This lineage is by no means complete. It is transcribed from Col. Chang's diagram (ca. 1974) and is simply presented here to show the relationship between Dennis Rovere, his teacher Col. Chang, and the contemporaries of Huang Bo Nien.

Huang was a student of Li Tsun-i (a contemporary of Sun Lu Tang). This therefore places him in the same generation as Col. Chang, the Chu brothers, et al. Because Li Li Rou and the Chu brothers were good friends, they are often placed in the same generation.

## ABOUT THE AUTHORS

DENNIS ROVERE is an internationally recognized expert in military close combat and Chinese military strategy. He is the first non-Asian to receive special recognition as a martial arts instructor from the Government of the Republic of China, and the first civilian to train with the Bodyguard Instructors' Unit of the Chinese Special Military Police (Wu Jing). Since receiving his instructor's certification in 1974, Mr. Rovere has taught martial arts to both civilians and military units, including reconnaissance instructors and UN peacekeepers. Rovere lives in Calgary, Canada with his wife, Chow Hon Huen, and their two children.

CHOW HON HUEN was born, raised, and educated in Hong Kong. This is her second martial art book translation; her first was *Chinese Military Police: Knife, Baton and Weapon Techniques,* also done in conjunction with Dennis Rovere.